Heart Family Handbook

Heart Family Handbook

A Complete Guide for the
Entire Family of Anyone
with Any Heart Condition—
to Help Make It the Speediest,
Most Complete Recovery Possible

Jane Schoenberg • **JoAnn Stichman**

HANLEY & BELFUS, INC.
Philadelphia

Publisher: HANLEY & BELFUS, INC.
210 S. 13th Street
Philadelphia, PA 19107
(215) 546-7293

This book is available at special discounts
with bulk purchases for educational purposes.
For further information, contact the publisher.

Part of the proceeds from this book will be
donated to the American Heart Association.

Heart Family Handbook
Library of Congress Catalog Card Number 89-81864
ISBN 0-932883-23-0

Printed in the United States of America
9 8 7 6 5 4 3 2 1

To our husbands, Arthur and Forrest; our children,
John and Peggy Stichman, Dennis and Kathy (Stichman) Adler,
David and Leslie Schoenberg, Eddie and Sharon Schoenberg,
Barton and Marcie (Schoenberg) Lee, and all the grandchildren

Contents

Introduction

Authors

For you, the most meaningful fact about us is that we know what you and your family are going through because we both went through it, and continue to do so. JoAnn's husband, Forrest, had a heart attack in 1964 at age 40; Jane's husband, Arthur, had a heart attack in 1966 at age 46.

Whenever we ran into each other during the late '60s, we eagerly compared notes about the problems of family adjustment to our husbands' long-term recoveries. We were the only people we knew in our age group who faced such problems; no one who had not gone through it seemed to understand.

Then, by a "coincidence" that's actually part of a pattern in families of heart patients, we met in a class at UCLA. Both of us had dropped out of college when we got married. We both, independently, decided to go back to school. You talk about "completing your education" and "fulfillment"; what you mean is, "Suppose he dies? How can I support the kids and myself if I don't have at least a college degree?"—a perfect example of the sorts of "unthinkable" things people in Heart Families do indeed think, though hardly ever say, then feel guilty about (see "Beauty Shop Problems" in chapter 7).

So when we both took a class that required a community service project, we teamed up to start "Heart Wives," a group that would formalize for others what we had long been doing for each other.

1

Between us, over the years, we have pretty well spanned the possibilities in Heart Family experience. Forrest Stichman made a marvelous recovery, with no recurrence. Arthur Schoenberg suffered three more heart attacks, had a bypass, was stricken with severe arrhythmias and congestive heart failure. Mere days away from death, in September 1986, he became, at age 66, the country's oldest heart transplant recipient. His recovery has been miraculous: he is now back at work—and golf!

Given our reasons for going back to school and the course of our husbands' heart conditions, our different occupations are significant. JoAnn has concentrated mostly on volunteer work: establishing the Heart Wife program at Cedars-Sinai Medical Center in Los Angeles, getting involved with the Women Helping Women hotline service, and with fund raising to shelter the homeless. Jane, whose activities before Arthur's first heart attack included such volunteer work as the presidency of The Associates of Vista Del Mar child care service, has since worked steadily at jobs with pay *and* insurance, first with her husband in their manufacturing business, then as administrative assistant to the head of pediatric nephrology at Children's Hospital and UCLA, and currently as editor for the UCLA Tissue-Typing Laboratory.

First Book

As a result of our experiences, we wrote *How to Survive Your Husband's Heart Attack* (David McKay Company, New York, 1974). *Survive* took the Heart Wife through all the adjustments she, her husband, and family must make to put their lives back together. It let her know she was not alone, showed what to expect, and what to do about it. *Survive* won the American Heart Association's Howard Blakeslee Award as the best heart book of 1974.

Heart Wife Program

The original group is still going, stronger than ever, at Cedars-Sinai. The term now used, however, is "Heart Family," an evolution with particular relevance to this book. A brochure promises the program will show "How your family can benefit from the experience and training of people who know how you feel."

The program has also started at other major coronary care centers across the country. The latest was at Houston's Baylor University Hospital, with a representative from the Cedars group dispatched to supervise the start-up.

This Book

A book like this has to help people cope by sharing experiences and allowing them to see that they're not the only people in the world who have gone through this.

It's also a very good opportunity to educate people about the current concepts of heart disease and what we're doing to treat the acute problems and deal with the aftermath.

—John Strobeck, M.D.

Of course that was the purpose of our first book, *Survive.* But Dr. Strobeck's "current concepts" make the coronary care of 1974 seem primitive. Furthermore, coronary disease has gone "equal opportunity," with ever larger numbers of women falling victim. At the same time, today's greater spirit of shared family responsibility affects health care. That's fortunate because, especially for today's many varieties and treatments of heart disease, family care is essential for complete recovery—which Dr. Hillel Laks, chief of cardiothoracic surgery at UCLA, defines as "getting back to a lifestyle *without* constant consciousness that one is ill, and not allowing illness to color one's activities and relationships."

How do patients reach that happy state? Dr. Laks continues: "Most patients are not really capable of achieving this kind of ideal lifestyle without a tremendous amount of support and motivation, which best comes from the family."

Plainly, our first book needed updating to include medical advances since 1974, to examine the entire family's role in helping the patient recover, and to explore ways the entire family could protect themselves against the hereditary heart disease that may well threaten the patient's children and siblings.

Can't all this information and support come from the professionals who treat the patient? Doctors and nurses are busy; patients and families often shy away from "bothering" starchy professionals. Even caring, sympathetic physicians like Dr. Frederick L. Grover, chief of cardiothoracic surgery at the Audie L. Murphy VA Hospital in San Antonio, are alert to the problem. "There are so many day-to-day questions," he says,

we physicians just can't sit down and spend enough time with the family. I realized that many years ago, and that's one reason I felt it very important to have a nurse coordinator help us—who can do this methodically. People may open up a little more to a nurse than to a doctor who comes through with two or three others on rounds. We don't give them a lot of opportunity for one-on-one.

But even the most conscientious nurse coordinator can't do the whole job. Dr. Grover continues:

> I think there's a special perspective that families who have been through an experience like this can offer that those of us in the profession can't—not even our coordinator. She goes into as much detail as she can about what to expect before and after surgery. Still, having someone who's been through it offers that extra perspective.

Not every hospital provides such thoughtful support—for lack of budget, resources, or interest. In any case, you and your family need that special perspective Dr. Grover mentioned. So whether you use this book as substitute or supplement, it will let you know that you are not alone, and will help you help your patient make the best, fastest, most complete recovery possible.

A few words on format. Entries within each chapter are presented in alphabetical order and are listed at the beginning of the chapter. At the start of Notes, in the back of the book, you'll find the titles and institutional affiliations of the health care professionals we quote by name; after the first mention we identify them in the text only when their specialty has some particular relevance to the passage. We identify in Notes any sources (including printed material) that we do not cite in the text. You'll find pertinent medical terms explained in the Glossary.

CHAPTER 1

The Difference Then and Now

Aggressive Treatment, Age of
Family, Role of the
Intervention
Rehabilitation

What's the difference in the heart disease situation between 1974, when *Survive* was published, and now?

The Introduction gave you the bad news that heart disease is up among women; the good news is that there is no more bad news. "The overall incidence of heart disease in the American population has decreased 27%," says Dr. Harvey Alpern, a Los Angeles cardiologist. This may strike you as the very definition of "cold comfort," since, despite statistics, someone in *your* family has a coronary problem. But consider a connected fact: "Over the last ten years," says Dr. Leon Resnekov, chief of cardiology at the University of Chicago, "there's been a progressive decline in *mortality* from coronary artery disease of 3% a year. So over one decade, we're down by almost one-third. It's very encouraging."

Most encouraging, and the best news of all, is the reason for both declines: the medical profession can do so much more for a patient. They detect heart problems earlier and treat them more effectively; they offer better long-term care and rehabilitation that includes better measures to prevent recurrence of problems. Furthermore, today's doctors and nurses have more help from greater numbers and a greater variety of health professionals, like dietitians and therapists, who know better how to help.

What was the situation before? Dr. Sam L. Teichman calls it "the Passive Age of Therapy" for heart disease. Once a practicing cardiologist, he now heads professional services at Genentech, a biopharmaceutical firm near San Francisco. In the Passive Age, Dr. Teichman points out, the "treatment" for heart attack was to put the

5

patient to bed for six weeks to three months, administering stool softeners so bowel movements wouldn't cause heart-taxing strain. Cardiologists would debate the wisdom of permitting the patient to sit up in bed on day 10—versus waiting until day 14. Now, many patients are *home* on day 7!

In the 1960s, with innovations like Coronary Care Units (CCUs) and the Swan-Ganz catheter, we entered what Dr. Teichman calls "the Reactive Age," a time "when complications were reacted to very rapidly and aborted"—arrhythmias checked, congestive conditions kept from becoming worse. "Still, the damage was done, and there was no intervention to abort or limit that damage."

Finally, in the late 1970s and early 1980s we entered today's "Aggressive Age." Now, doctors do intervene; they forestall, abort, even reverse the course of a heart attack. And the picture gets rosier all the time. "Over the past 10 years," says Dr. William C. DeVries, the surgeon who performed the world's first human artificial heart implant, "we've virtually exploded technologically. I remember how difficult it was in 1975, even 1979, to do surgery. I remember having to tell patients, 'You've got a one out of four chance of dying tomorrow.' Now I'm talking 99 out of 100 doing fine—no problems at all. And the horizon is really unlimited."

Aggressive Treatment, Age of

Carole Landers, R.N., manager of the rehabilitation center at the Humana Heart Institute, International in Louisville, remembers that in 1975 patients routinely stayed in a CCU, flat on their backs, for at least seven days. Now, in seven days, as noted above, they may be home, and the rehab people are likely to have them pumping away on a stationary bike in two weeks.

"The treatment for heart attack is never just 'Go to bed for six weeks' any more," says Dr. Lawrence H. Cohn, chief of cardiac surgery at Boston's Brigham & Women's Hospital. "We're out of that realm completely; we're into a totally activist approach: the combination of these thrombolytic agents and the balloons and surgery and all this. It is saving lives, no question."

Family, Role of the

A doctor we talked with gives the best validation of the family's part in aggressive intervention and rehabilitation. "Some patients," he says, "have no family—and they're the hardest ones to deal with!"

Intervention

Intervention is the key to treatment for all coronary problems today. It is no longer a question of, as one doctor puts it, "everyone standing with fingers crossed, hoping for a favorable outcome." Today's doctors can intervene in the course of heart disease. They dissolve blood clots and restore flow to the heart muscle, open clogged arteries, surgically bypass the blockage in closed arteries, repair leaky valves. They can stop the heart from beating irregularly.

Maybe even more important, doctors and other health care professionals now intervene in the course of coronary disease itself, retarding, even preventing, its development, before *and* after such coronary incidents as heart attacks and angina. Certain risk factors (see chapter 2) once were thought "beyond control"—such as a disposition to high cholesterol. But, as one doctor says, "if we can drive the cholesterol level far below normal, we are intervening, somewhat, even in the genetic aspect."

How to help the professionals intervene, and make the most of their intervention, is the message of this book.

Rehabilitation (Also see Chapter 11)

Little in coronary care has changed as dramatically as the concept of rehabilitation—getting patients back as soon as possible to the level of pre-treatment activity, and, at the same time, changing behavior to affect risk factors favorably.

A hospital-run rehab program typically starts two or three weeks after discharge. The rehab staff evaluates the condition and stamina of new clients (rehab people carefully avoid saying "patients"). Then they design a course of exercise that steadily increases the amount of exertion required, monitoring the client's heart all the way. In addition, clients will talk with dietitians and stress management therapists who steer them toward modification of behavior patterns that increased the risk of heart disease *for that individual.*

The University of Ottawa Heart Institute's Prevention and Rehabilitation Centre at the Ottawa Civic Hospital, directed by Dr. William Dafoe, pursues a multi-dimensional comprehensive approach to rehabilitation. Their staff includes nurses, physiotherapists, vocational rehabilitation counsellors, a social worker, psychologist, dietitian, and occupational therapist.

Staff nurse Patti Robbins assesses those entering the program, then functions as a coordinator for the individual's program. In addition to the care offered by team members, she views a client's understanding of his own responsibility for rehabilitation as an important ingredient for eventual change.

With most programs, clients attend three 1-hour rehab sessions a week for somewhere between 8 and 12 weeks (in Ottawa, 6 months). After that, they continue their own rehab at home, exercising bodies and, equally important, exercising their wills and intellects to build a saner way of living for themselves and their families.

"We try," says Karen Krozek, R.N., a rehab specialist in Santa Monica, California, "to give them a lot of facts, which means continued education on *living* with heart disease. The original cause may not lie in any one particular risk factor; but it's been shown over and over again that the lifestyle habits we have can contribute to heart disease or, by the same token, forestall it. So we make clients aware that they do have a lot of control over what happens to their hearts; and we give them tools to change."

CHAPTER 2

Heart Conditions:
What's Wrong and Why

How the Heart Works and
   What Can Go Wrong
Angina Pectoris
Arrhythmia
Cardiomyopathy

Congestive Heart Failure
Heart Attack (Coronary Occlusion/
   Myocardial Infarction)
Valves
What They All Have in Common

We try to provide patients with as much basic information and insight
as possible into the natural history of their coronary disease: "if you
don't do *anything* you may be around ten years from now"; what's the
response to medication; what are the possibilities of surgery. That's to
help them weigh the risks and benefits of the possible courses of
treatment.

We try to do it not just with the patient but with the spouse and
other members of the family. The more the family understands, the
better they're able to help the patient.

—Dr. Allan M. Lansing
Director
Humana Heart Institute, International
Louisville

What You Should Know First—Even If It Is Out Of Alphabetical Order: How the Heart Works and What Can Go Wrong

Most of us start with only the dimmest notion of what causes a
heart attack, let alone more obscure conditions such as cardiomyopathy. That may seem strange, considering how much we hear
about heart disease these days. But most of the talk is directed to
things like telling us to quit smoking and to watch our cholesterol—
or to selling us polyunsaturated margarine, aspirin, and oat bran. Yet
unless we understand the mechanics of a failing heart, how can we

9

help the patient avoid future problems? And unless we comprehend the vocabulary of heart disease, we cannot hope to understand what the doctors and nurses are telling us about our patient's particular problem.

All heart conditions come down to this: something is making it difficult or impossible for the heart to pump blood throughout the body. The heart is a very strong muscle. Every time it "beats" it contracts, squeezing itself so that the blood inside its two lower chambers (ventricles) is forced out. The blood in the right ventricle, which lacks oxygen, goes to the lungs for a resupply. The blood in the left ventricle, its red cells charged with oxygen by the lungs, carries that oxygen to tissue throughout the body.

When the heart relaxes, after each contraction, the lowered pressure pulls blood into the two upper chambers (atria—the Latin plural of atrium). The blood filling the right atrium comes from veins all over the body, depleted of oxygen; the blood filling the left atrium comes from the lungs, newly charged with oxygen.

A wall of muscle (septum) separates the right and left sides of the heart. Two valves connect the atria and ventricles; two more separate the ventricles and the arteries they push blood into. The four valves open and close in rhythm so that blood flows only in the useful directions: from the atria to the ventricles, from the ventricles to the arteries. If anything interferes with this pavan of contracting and relaxing, of opening and closing, or if anything impedes the free flow of blood, the body finds itself in some degree of trouble. Any tissue that gets no blood (and so no oxygen) dies. Tissue that does not get enough blood may not die, but will certainly get "sick," and report the abuse by producing pain.

So anything called "heart disease" is simply some condition that in some manner interferes with the proper flow of blood in the proper quantity.

Now you're ready to look at the particular condition that afflicts *your* patient.

Angina Pectoris*

The heart pumps oxygen-bearing blood to all tissue in the body. The more work tissue does, the more oxygen it needs. Since the heart

---

* This is the full, formal name, "pectoris" being Latin for "of the breast," "angina" deriving from a Greek word meaning "throttling," because of the "tight" feeling in the chest, a characteristic symptom. The malady's acquaintances (it has no friends) call it simply "angina."

is muscle tissue, and since it works harder than any other muscle (each day beating about 100,000 times, pumping some 2,000 gallons of blood), it needs more blood than most other tissue. Sensibly, the heart feeds itself first by way of the two coronary arteries, the first to branch off from the aorta, the main artery out of the heart (see illustration section following page 16). Each coronary artery runs about four to five inches, with many branches that reach all parts of the heart. At its widest, the opening (lumen) in a coronary artery is about one-eighth of an inch across—which may not sound very wide, but is actually more than enough, the word "more" being extremely important because coronary arteries have a nasty habit of clogging. A fatty substance called cholesterol tends to cling to the inner lining of the artery, irritating the lining. The body automatically covers any irritation with tough, fibrous scar tissue. More cholesterol accumulates, then more fiber, layer on layer, along with whatever stray cells happen along, a mixture called "plaque." The lumen keeps narrowing.

Until the artery is about 70% narrowed, no sign of trouble exists; indeed, some people with arterial openings less than 10% experience no pain. But for most, angina develops—a matter of supply and demand. Sit with your legs firmly crossed for long enough, and one leg will "fall asleep." Pressure on the main artery feeding your leg has pinched it, reducing blood supply to tissue below the pressure point, starving that tissue of oxygen. The painful sensation is tissue's way of telling you to cut it out before tissue starts to die. But remember that the more exertion, the more oxygen tissue needs. So you would get the same result—the familiar "athlete's cramp"—with exercise violent beyond reason.

That describes exactly what happens with the heart, its coronary arteries, and angina. The pain usually comes from a combination of lowered blood supply through narrowed arteries and the increased demand of exercise.

Even when plaque narrows the artery by, say, 80%, the supply of blood getting through is enough to perfuse the heart tissue adequately as long as it's doing nothing much. Ask the heart to pump harder—to feed the rest of the body's tissue while it plays tennis or golf or runs or, maybe, just walks up stairs—and, like the tissue it supplies, the heart, too, needs more blood. A narrowed coronary artery cannot meet the demand. The oxygen-starved heart tissue signifies its distress in the usual manner, by hurting, warning the patient to stop putting the extra, unmeetable demand on it.

Exercise isn't the only trigger. Nerve-stretching stress, tooth-grinding tension, the degree of emotion novelists would call "heart-pounding"—all cause the heart to beat a tattoo, demanding extra blood that the clogged artery cannot supply. What's more, if anything further constricts a narrowed artery, even temporarily, supply falls short of demand. Spasms, whose cause are unknown, can do it. So can smoking.

Most anginas are stable, their symptoms and the amount of exertion that will trigger them staying the same, often for years. When they become unstable—for instance, when pain occurs with increasingly less exertion, or even without exertion—the situation (which may well have been under good medical control) becomes serious. Unstable angina figures to become heart attack, and that calls for dramatic intervention.

Arrhythmia

When everything's working as it should, a group of cells called "the sinus node" in the right atrium sparks a bit of electricity that travels through both atria, causing them to contract, forcing their blood into their respective ventricles. This happens a scant moment before the electric signal pulses throughout both ventricles over a network of special conductive fibers, causing the ventricles to contract.

It's a symphony of timing, regular and rhythmic.

The beat can change three ways. The sinus node may spark too fast or too slowly; something can cause a blockage in the wiring system that carries the signal; abnormalities in heart tissue can make different parts of the heart set their own tempo of contraction. Many factors can set off these irregularities, most of them commonplace, with relatively benign results—the way too much coffee sets some perfectly normal hearts racing (tachycardia) or makes them skip a beat (premature ventricular contraction, PVC).

Irritation of heart tissue—let alone a full-scale heart attack—can bring on arrhythmias, which can be desperately serious. About 50% of deaths due to heart attacks happen in the first hour, almost all the result of arrhythmias, the most fearsome and common being ventricular tachycardia and ventricular fibrillation. In tachycardia, the ventricle sets its own pounding beat, a beat so inefficient that little blood escapes the aorta. Fibrillation is the real killer, though, with the ventricle not really contracting but merely twitching; blood flow, pulse, and breathing completely stop, with death imminent unless someone quickly halts the fibrillation. Doctors call this condition "cardiac arrest."

Cardiomyopathy*

The two basic forms of cardiomyopathy share the mournful distinction of being intractable to really effective treatment. Furthermore, with one exception, their causes are unknown, what doctors call "idiopathic,"† although too much alcohol may trigger it.

In the more usual form, the heart muscle itself swells, which means that it stretches, thins, and therefore grows weaker as the size of the heart grows. The left ventricle no longer pumps blood efficiently, resulting in congestive heart failure and, sometimes, blood clots that block other arteries, causing strokes.

The other form of the disease sees a thickening of the wall of the left ventricle and sometimes the septum separating the two ventricles. The symptoms of this form are generally less severe.

Congestive Heart Failure

When the heart muscle, especially that of the left ventricle, becomes so damaged, or so much of it has died, that it lacks the strength to keep blood flowing with anything like normal efficiency, blood and other body fluids start to back up throughout the body, a congestion.

Swelling (edema) results, especially in the ankles and legs. If fluid congests the lungs, a patient can hardly breathe; it's like drowning. And since none of the backed up blood or fluid carries oxygen, and the damaged ventricle delivers less oxygen-rich blood, the body weakens. The kidneys fail to eliminate water, which further increases edema and the burden on the heart.

Continued long enough, this process shuts down circulation, a usually fatal condition called "cardiogenic shock."

The three causes of congestive heart failure are severe or repeated heart attacks, heart valves that don't work right, and chronic high blood pressure.

Heart Attack (Coronary Occlusion/Myocardial Infarction)‡

If plaque continues to clog a coronary artery (see "Angina," above), the flow of blood eventually will be entirely blocked. Before

---

* Literally derived from Greek, "heart muscle suffering."

† A learned-sounding way of saying, "We just don't know." The "pathy" part, same as in "cardiomyopathy," means "suffering"; "idio" is a form of the Greek for "one's own" or "separate," as in "idiosyncratic."

‡ See footnote on page 14.

that, though, a blood clot usually forms at the plaque-narrowed spot, suddenly shutting off the barely adequate trickle. A spasm (cause unknown) may also constrict an artery already so narrowed by plaque that, again, it suddenly shuts altogether.

However it happens, the result is the same. Tissue "down stream" of the blockage gets no more blood, so no more oxygen. It starts to die. Once dead, that heart muscle tissue can no longer contract and relax in heart beat.

Dying takes heart tissue four to six hours, but the shock may cause ventricular fibrillation (see "Arrhythmias," above), which may end in sudden death from cardiac arrest.

As with angina, oxygen-starved tissue protests by causing pain—how much depending on how much heart muscle is affected. If blockage occurs in only a minor coronary branch, the pain may be insignificant, mistaken for mere indigestion or ignored altogether; doctor's call this a "silent heart attack."

Like pain, the severity of the heart attack depends on how much heart muscle is affected, and which parts. A patient can readily survive an attack that destroys much right ventricle tissue, while blockage of the left main coronary artery, feeding the left ventricle, is usually fatal.

Incidentally, cocaine can so constrict coronary arteries that instant, total blockage takes place.

After three days, or thereabouts, even if no one has done anything to stem its effects, a heart attack has caused all the short-term physical damage *that* attack is going to cause.

Valves

The four coronary valves are made of flexible, tough flaps of tissue. If normal, they are easily pushed open by a flow of blood in the right direction, forced shut by any flow the wrong way (see illustration section following page 16). However, a few circumstances, generally the ravages of rheumatic fever or congenital deformities, can so distort the flaps (called "leaflets" or "cusps") that they either cannot open or cannot close completely.

---

‡ Not exactly synonyms. "Occlusion," from the Latin for "to shut," refers to the complete blocking of a coronary artery. That leads to infarction of the myocardium ("heart muscle" in Latinized Greek). By "infarction," doctors mean severe damage or death; but the word comes directly from the Latin for "stuffed" (kin to the French cookery term *farcie*, as well as "forcemeat" and "farce"). That suggests the process of occlusion rather than its result. Did the doctors get hold of the wrong word?

When a valve cannot open fully ("stenosis" or "narrowed valve"), not enough blood goes through; blood backs up, causing undue pressure in the never-quite-emptied chamber. When a valve cannot fully close ("leaky valve"), blood goes through, then flows partly back in the wrong direction (coronary "regurgitation" or "insufficiency"), forcing the heart to pump harder to get enough blood in circulation. Some valves suffer both problems.

A heart laboring to overcome valve problems weakens. Often, it becomes distorted in size to compensate. That works well for a while, but eventually the situation degenerates; for example, valve problems can induce congestive heart failure.

What They All Have in Common

Many of the diseases that afflict us are potentially much more dangerous than most heart conditions, especially considering the dramatic progress in treatment we'll examine in chapter 4. Once you are over such potential killers as tuberculosis, typhus, typhoid, and pulmonary pneumonia, you have no more reason to fear those diseases than before you got them. Your own life need not be particularly different; your family need make no special adjustments. That's true even with cancer, five years after successful treatment. You might say those diseases can kill you, but they can't hurt you.

Any heart condition is different; all differ in the same way. No "cure" exists. The *condition* that caused the condition persists and remains essentially ineradicable. Another onset can come at any time, with no sure way to prevent it. The patient can, however, do certain things to slash the chances of recurrence, and those things amount to a different sort of life for the patient, spouse, indeed the entire family—still with no guarantees. People can be careful, do all the right things . . . and drop dead tomorrow. Think what it means to live with that!

"People with coronary conditions are different from any other patients," says one cardiologist. "It's almost as though they go through a grieving process for something they've lost, something that strikes at what they perceive as the core of their existence."

If they had a heart attack, they probably experienced severe pain, knew mortal peril. Even "saved," they face a future that can always hold more pain and sudden death. They don't know if they will be able to work as hard or as well as before. Or at all. Will they be able to earn as much as before? Take care of their family as well? Can they now hope ever to achieve their former goals? They'll have to stop smoking, watch their weight, give up many foods, maybe some activities, they enjoyed. Most important, will they be the people they had always thought themselves?

"The heart condition," continues the same doctor, "can affect a person psychologically much more than anything else. But it's hard to know how any individual is going to react. Some don't react right away; maybe denial prevents them from reacting. Then, when they're presumably 'better,' they begin to deal with it, begin to react. It's very confusing to the family."

That, of course, is one of the principal reasons for this book. Now let's see what can be done about all the conditions we've looked at.

Illustrations

The following illustrations are reproduced with permission from *Heart Beat* by Emmanuel Horovitz, M.D., Health Trend Publishing, P.O. Box 17420, Encino, CA 91416, © 1988 by Emmanuel Horovitz, M.D.

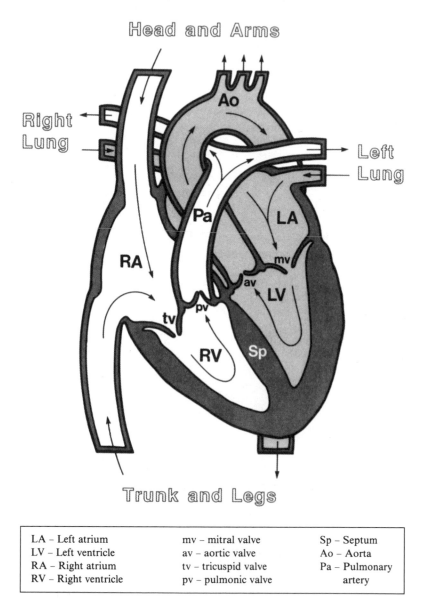

LA – Left atrium	mv – mitral valve	Sp – Septum
LV – Left ventricle	av – aortic valve	Ao – Aorta
RA – Right atrium	tv – tricuspid valve	Pa – Pulmonary
RV – Right ventricle	pv – pulmonic valve	artery

Figure 1. The heart chambers, heart valves, major blood vessels, and circulatory system.

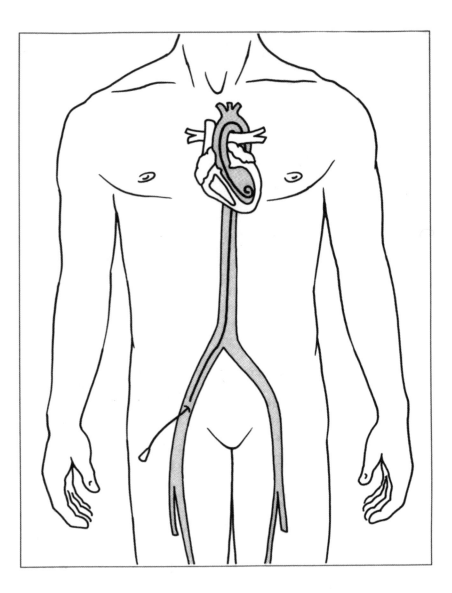

Figure 2. During cardiac catheterization, a catheter is inserted into a peripheral artery (or vein) and then directed toward the heart. Here, the tip of the catheter is shown inside the left ventricle.

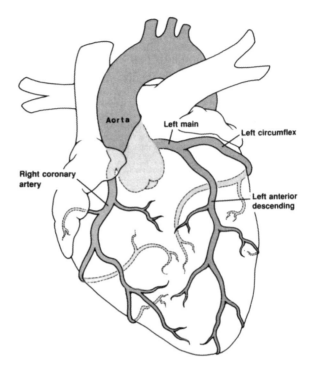

Figure 3. The coronary arteries.

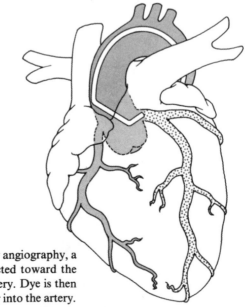

Figure 4. During coronary angiography, a pre-shaped catheter is directed toward the opening of the coronary artery. Dye is then injected through the catheter into the artery.

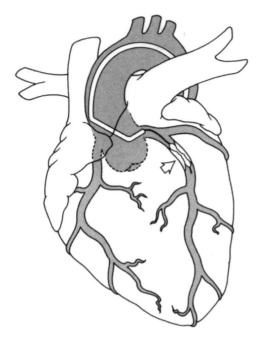

Figure 5. Coronary balloon angioplasty. The guiding catheter is directed toward the opening of the coronary artery. The thinner dilatation catheter is then threaded through the guiding catheter and advanced into the coronary artery, until the balloon reaches the area of narrowing.

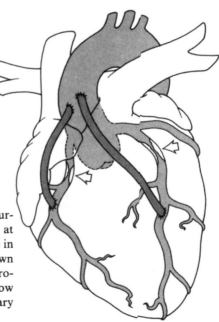

Figure 6. Coronary bypass surgery. The vein graft is attached at one end to a small opening made in the aorta, and the other end is sewn to an opening created in the coronary artery. Blood can now flow from the aorta into the coronary artery, beyond the blockage.

CHAPTER 3

How It Got That Way (Risk Factors)

Age

Cholesterol

Diabetes

Diet

Exercise, Lack of

Gender

Guilty, Save Time: Plead

Heredity

High Blood Pressure

Smoking

Stress

Whole Family, Implications for

> *Mrs. A:* They said it was mild heart attack, "a random clot"; they didn't know how or why it happened; his mother swears it was the humidity—and because my husband "didn't eat enough nourishing cream."
>
> *Heart Wife Counselor:* My mother was sure it was because my husband drove the freeways.
>
> *Mrs. A:* We all have our theories, but we'll never know why . . .

Age

Not that anyone can do anything about it, but the older you get, the greater your risk of heart disease. Plaque has longer to build up; valves become misshapen. Sadly, though, more younger people become afflicted nowadays. "In this area of country," says a doctor in New Jersey, "we see a lot of people in their thirties with heart attacks. The youngest I've seen so far with a non-drug–related heart attack was 26." No one can account for the drop in age, although one therapist guesses that stress is more widespread now.

Cholesterol (Also see "Diet," below)

"I think the cholesterol question today is where smoking was in 1970," says Mary Bowlby, a dietitian at the University of Ottawa Heart

Institute Prevention and Rehabilitation Centre at the Ottawa Civic Hospital. The statistical evidence of connection between high cholesterol and heart disease has become so weighty that nearly everyone recognizes the danger, despite a continuing lack of proof that one *causes* the other.

The only room for doubt lies in the fact that the cholesterol clogging arteries is never the cholesterol we eat. The body needs cholesterol, a soft, fatty substance. Cells make their membranes, vitamin D, and sex hormones from it; they use it to protect nerve fibers. But the cholesterol they use is manufactured mostly by the liver, and made almost entirely from other fats and carbohydrates, not whatever cholesterol we eat.

You can understand the problem researchers had tagging eaten cholesterol a villain. Consume only 1 milligram of cholesterol, and that's all your liver needs for a day's production. In fact, most Americans gobble up more than 600 milligrams a day. Still, no one could point to a single molecule of eaten cholesterol that ended up as arterial plaque. By now, though, researchers have conducted enough studies to convince the most skeptical: the more cholesterol and saturated fat you eat, the more cholesterol the liver produces, which means the higher the cholesterol level in the blood, the more likely you are to have heart disease. As with the connection between smoking and heart disease (and, of course, cancer), no doubt lingers among medical people.

Diabetes

Without knowing quite how it happens, doctors assure us that those with diabetes are more apt to develop atherosclerosis, especially if uncontrolled. Maybe high blood sugar promotes higher cholesterol levels, or diabetics tend to be overweight and have high blood pressure, two more risk factors. Whatever the mechanics, the only thing heart patients and their families really have to know about diabetes is summed up by one distinguished cardiologist who says, flatly, "It's *important* to control."

Diet

Start with the extreme problem. The heart of an obese person has to work almost twice as hard as the heart of someone at normal weight. Even short of obesity, bad diet becomes a heart problem. First, a diet high in fats, specifically saturated fat and cholesterol (see above), raises the cholesterol level in the blood, with attendant risk of heart disease. Diets high in sodium lead to fluid retention and high blood pressure.* That is of mortal importance for anyone who has already demonstrated a heart problem.

Exercise, Lack of

Lack of exercise is not, strictly speaking, a risk factor; no one has drawn a convincing link between *not* exercising and developing any form of heart disease. Instead, exercising is what you might call an "anti-risk factor." "Two studies," a cardiologist tells us, "indicate a lower incidence of heart disease with regular aerobic exercise." Equally important, exercise makes the heart better able to withstand the ravages of any attack that does happen.

Exercise can also help reduce overweight, an unquestioned risk factor. A Stanford University study shows that although dieting and exercise each can help take off weight, pounds lost through exercise are purely fat, while dieters may shed muscle, leaving them weaker.

Exercise also cuts levels of cholesterol and triglycerides and raises the level of high-density lipoproteins, the so-called "good cholesterol" (see "Cholesterol" in chapter 4).

So, although sitting about won't bring on heart disease, exercise almost surely prevents or retards it.

Gender

Another uncontrollable factor. Despite the upswing in heart disease among women in the past decade, until age 65, men are still about twice as likely to be afflicted. Doctors think that the presence of female hormones retards the buildup of plaque, although they can't imagine how or why.

Guilty, Save Time: Plead

Three kinds of guilt attach themselves to heart conditions. The first is religious. Dr. William Dafoe at the University of Ottawa Heart Institute Prevention and Rehabilitation Centre at the Ottawa Civic Hospital relates an example of this kind, in which "a young lady with very strict Catholic upbringing felt a tremendous amount of guilt,

---

* Salt is the most common form of sodium, but as a glance at the label of nearly any canned food will show you, forms of sodium are the usual food preservatives. See chapter 9 for details.

thinking it was her own fault she had a heart problem." She considered it divine punishment. The doctor arranged for her to talk with a priest who understood the medical as well as spiritual ramifications, and could reassure her that one did not derive from the other.

The other two kinds of guilt are secular.

First comes the guilt of patients who feel, "Look what I have done to my family, the misery I may cause if I die—and maybe even greater misery if I live and am a burden or cannot take care of them the way I used to; and all because I didn't take care of myself." All these self-reproaches can afflict men and women equally.

The third kind of guilt, shared by family members, changes slightly depending on age and sex. One woman rushed to meet the cardiologist as he emerged from the Coronary Care Unit after examining her husband the first time. Yes, it was a heart attack, but her husband would be all right. Radiating relief, she asked what she could do to help in his recovery. "Get that fat off him," the doctor snapped, leaving her feeling, she says, "like a naughty little girl who was too dumb, or too lazy, to have done her duty."

Similarly, dietitian Mary Bowlby reports that the guilt she finds hardest to deal with is the guilt that comes with being told as the wife of the patient about to be discharged "to watch his cholesterol," when in fact she thought she'd been doing a wonderful job all along—and, in fact, had been! "When that happens," Bowlby observes, "the person who is upset is not the patient, it's the wife, especially in the generation where a woman's whole raison d'être was to be the care-giver, the person who made the meals and made healthy families and so on. To be told, now, when you're 65, that you blew it is a kick in the face."

Bowlby tries to convince such self-accusers that diet may not have had anything to do with the case, that heredity may also figure strongly in cholesterol levels. "It takes," she says, "a lot of convincing."

With men it can take even more. How do you convince someone like Mr. G. who feels guilty that he did not take a stronger hand when his wife's condition was first diagnosed many years ago, insisting that she do the things that might have corrected or palliated the condition before it became a heart attack, requiring a bypass operation that has left her, essentially, a cardiac cripple. He berates himself for not having played the more manly part, overcoming what he recognized as his wife's inertia. "Twenty years ago I should have pushed her more," he says, "and I don't think she would have had the heart attack. But you don't do that with Barbara. So I can't blame myself— at least I shouldn't blame myself—because you can only push so far. But I do feel bad and guilty. . . ."

Children of all ages, but especially the young ones living at home, can be haunted by fear that something they did caused it all. Giving a hard time, maybe? Not paying enough mind? Did that bring on mom's or dad's condition?

Allaying all three kinds of guilt takes a lot of convincing.

"I try to make them understand one of the basics," says Albert McClure, R.N., a clinical coordinator at Humana in Louisville, liaison with families of coronary surgical patients. "It's not something they or their spouses have done in the last 10 months or even 10 years, probably; it takes a long time to bring on the condition being treated. That's where we start."

Furthermore, it's never any one thing; it's an accumulation of risk factors, some of which are beyond anyone's control. Remember how often we've noted that little is known about how a particular condition develops or what, exactly, causes it. Ponder the results of a number of studies into the cause of heart disease.

Stress is a risk factor (see "Stress," below), and soldiers in combat surely face a nearly intolerable amount of it. During the Korean War, army doctors performed autopsies on 300 American soldiers killed in action. Their age averaged just over 22, yet more than three-quarters evidenced heart disease, some with branch arteries completely clogged. Was stress the cause? Unlikely, because matching autopsies on Chinese soldiers, who were obviously under the same stress, revealed almost no heart disease. Doctors had conducted similar studies after World War II among prisoners who survived Nazi concentration camps, and among citizens of Stalingrad, a city under siege for over two years. Those people had lived under stress as nerve-wracking as combat, and for a lot longer. Yet autopsies on those who died of whatever cause disclosed virtually no heart disease among them!

Stress seemed not to matter. But consider diet. Our soldiers ate what most of us eat: foods high in fat content. The Chinese soldiers at mostly rice, vegetables, maybe some fish. The prisoners and the people of Stalingrad ate practically nothing (many starved to death), certainly not much meat, no dairy products at all. Autopsies on those who died shortly after the end of their terrifying experience showed that fatty deposits in the coronary arteries had been absorbed by the body, which devoured every ounce of available fat. Six months after the war, heart attacks again struck in Stalingrad and among the ex-prisoners. And the coronary disease rate in these groups soon climbed back to prewar levels.

So the most important factor in heart disease must be diet, right?

Then how about the survey made among some 31,000 employees of the London Transport Authority? Conductors on double-decker buses had significantly less heart disease than did the rest, including drivers and, significantly, conductors on single-deckers. All these men presumably ate pretty much the same things. Perhaps the double-decker conductors labored under less strain than their drivers, but no less than single-deck conductors. In fact, researchers identified the only real difference among the 31,000: the low-coronary disease group got more exercise than the others, tramping up and down the stairs of their double-deckers all day long.

Is regular exercise the key, then? A survey conducted by two teams—one in Boston, the other in Dublin—might seem to confirm that. Doctors studied 575 pairs of brothers. One of each pair had emigrated as a young man to the Boston area; the other brother stayed in Ireland. The results, after nine years of study, amazed the researchers. The Irishmen, as a group, had far less heart disease than their American brothers, even though the Irish brothers ate from 400 to 500 calories a day more, including a substantially higher percentage of animal fats, rich in the dreaded cholesterol! The difference: they mostly still worked their farms and in general got way more exercise.

Does that settle it? Not a bit. Swedish doctors conducted a similar study involving 32 pairs of identical twins, only one of whom had had a heart attack. After exhaustive testing, only one significant difference between the pairs emerged: those twins who had suffered heart attacks worked harder (though not at physical labor), relaxed less, had more personal, home, and business problems, and in general enjoyed life less. That adds up to . . . stress. Which brings us full circle.

Sensible people can reasonably come to only four conclusions: heart conditions take a long time to develop; they result from a combination of risk factors; some of the factors remain beyond anyone's control; no one can possibly say which one or combination of factors precipitated *this* person's condition.

But let's say that somehow you could be sure improper diet caused a particular condition—and you're primarily responsible for providing family meals. Are you guilty? You can prepare meals for them, but you can't eat for them. And you exercise little or no control over what they eat outside.

Or suppose that Mr. G. had kept after his wife to take better care of herself. Then if she'd had a heart attack anyway (suggestively, her mother had suffered one at a relatively early age), he could have tortured himself that the stress of his constant nag, nag, nag brought it on.

Well, if nothing you can do will assure immunity, and, worse, if you can hold yourself responsible whether you did or failed to do some things doctors say can at least help prevent heart conditions—

if therefore you cannot escape feeling guilty no matter what you did or didn't do—then what real meaning can the words "responsible" and "guilty" have in this situation?

So why do we tell you to save time and plead guilty?

Two reasons. First, everything above is rational, and when someone is stricken with a heart condition, experience proves that the person routinely feels guilty about having inflicted that on the family and the family feels guilty for either having caused it or not having done something to prevent it. Rationality plays no part in those judgments.

More important, your supposed "guilt" simply does not matter. Only what you do from here on out counts. Even if your guilt feelings have substance, surely the best contrition would be to do everything possible to prevent recurrence. That's the purpose of this book: to help families help the patient make the best, fastest recovery possible, with optimal rehabilitation. When you understand the risk factors, you can help avoid them in the future for the person already stricken and, equally important, for the rest of the family.

You still get no guarantees. If things turn out badly, you may feel the same irrational guilt you face now. But if you have done your best to reduce all known and controllable risks of heart disease, all you really feel guilt about is the unfortunate fact that you are human and not perfect.

Heredity

Heredity is another uncontrollable factor—except for the happy news you'll find in "Cholesterol," in chapter 4. A disposition toward high levels of cholesterol and high blood pressure, and indeed toward heart attacks (the sum of the risks) seems to run in families.

Unlike the other two uncontrollable risk factors, age and gender, this one bears serious implications for the whole family that the whole family most surely can control (see "Whole Family," below).

High Blood Pressure (Hypertension)

"Blood pressure" means the pressure of blood against the walls of the arteries it flows through, that pressure caused by the heart's pumping. The arteries—especially the smaller branches, called "arterioles"—resist the flow of blood, expanding to accommodate it. If they lose their elasticity, resistance goes up, and the heart must work harder to force blood through the arteries.

When pressure is up, a number of things may happen, all of them bad, including damage to the brain, kidneys, and eyes. In terms of heart disease, two terrible results may follow: (1) the heart may enlarge, working its way through inefficiency toward congestive heart failure; (2) plaque may build up faster in arteries under high blood pressure, speeding the time of occlusion. "If you don't control high blood pressure," one cardiologist explains, "you're almost *guaranteed* to have a heart attack, and/or a stroke. Control it and your risk drops *way* down." Fortunately, it is relatively simple to control, as we'll see in chapter 4.

Doctors do not know what causes over 90% of cases of high blood pressure,* which makes it hard to prevent. But serious overweight, undue stress, and too much salt in the diet seem related to the progress of the disease.

Smoking

Do we really need this section? Do you really have to read it? By now, anyone who maintains that the statistical correlation between smoking and heart disease (not to mention cancer) is coincidental, or that smoking causes nothing worse than holes in polyester clothing— that person has a mind fit only for creating tobacco company advertisements.

"Smoking is clearly associated with heart attacks," one cardiologist flatly declares. It damages the walls of the coronary arteries; the carbon dioxide smoking introduces into the bloodstream raises the level of fatty acids and helps fatty substances penetrate arterial walls, which may promote the buildup of plaque. Moreover, smoking constricts blood vessels and cuts the supply of oxygen to body tissue. In all, smoking doubles the risk of heart attack and may increase the risk of sudden death four times. Add smoking to high blood pressure and high cholesterol, and the risk of developing heart disease increases by ten.

A cardiac surgeon in Texas calls a failure to quit smoking "just crazy," and says about heart transplant candidates, "we won't operate on someone who hasn't demonstrated the ability to stop smoking." Donors are too rare. When doctors get a heart for transplant, he says, "it has to go to somebody who will take care of himself." At the University of Ottawa Heart Institute, smokers have three months to quit or they must leave the rehabilitation program.

We end with the American Heart Association's cry, just as it's printed: "STOP SMOKING NOW!"

---

* They call this kind of hypertension "essential," kissing cousin to "idiopathic."

Stress

Researchers know stress can generate heart disease: they have seen it happen in controlled experiments with monkeys. They know what happens: stress causes the brain to release hormones that prepare the body to fight or flee; the heart beats harder; arteries constrict. If it happens regularly and severely enough the arteries are damaged, and arterial damage sooner or later ends in atherosclerosis.

Two problems exist. "One problem with stress is that it's an integral part of life," says the head of cardiology at a big, city hospital. "I don't know how you can eliminate that unless you stop living. Take an executive. Stress is part of that job. So, unless he's going to change that job, he cannot avoid some stress." Besides, as one rehabilitation specialist points out, "we'd be dull people without some stress to keep us going."

The other problem is determining what constitutes stress for a particular person. You cannot simply say that astronauts and police face stress that could precipitate heart disease while ditchdiggers and afghan-makers don't. In the first place, as one doctor who addressed the subject wrote, "Some people . . . thrive on stress; they find working under pressure or against deadlines highly stimulating." Then, too, the afghan-maker who yearns to be a cop may sit crocheting with teeth clenched, suffused with the considerable stress of what Thoreau called "a life of quiet desperation."

The trick is to help particular people with heart conditions evaluate the level of stress they face, and help figure out what to do about lowering it.

Whole Family, Implications for the

"My viewpoint about heart disease is slightly different from that of most people," says Dr. Shahbudin Rahimtoola, chief of cardiology at County/USC Medical Center in Los Angeles.

When a parent has a heart attack, it signals to the family that the children are at greater risk. It's a matter of the family beginning to look at itself, a warning that the family should do something to correct risk factors—a change of lifestyle in the offspring.

So that heart attack really has enormously more long-term implications for the children than it has for the patient and spouse.

In some families it is not hard to make the connection. Mrs. A's 12-year-old son has some congenital heart problems, so his father's heart attack particularly devastated him. "It was like, 'Oh, my God, my father!'" says Mrs. A. "He saw this person whom he had considered perfectly healthy having this heart attack, and thinking, 'Oh, my God, I could be next!'" Indeed he could, even without the already identified congenital heart problems. Dr. Leon Resnekov, head of cardiology at the University of Chicago, talking about research on cholesterol and other lipid* abnormalities, says,

> Once you wish to apply what you've learned about these things at the research bench, the only way to do it logically is to involve the whole family.
>
> It's not simply that husband, Joe, has to have some special food prepared for him by his wife. We're very much interested in children. These processes begin at birth or even before birth, since these blood-fat abnormalities are really genetically determined; they're present at birth. You can see the problems already starting in coronary arteries of infants who happen to die of some other cause and autopsies are done. You see exactly where the problems are going to be many years down the road.

Of course the stricken person has to forge a new lifestyle anyway, and even if we shortsightedly ignore the implications for the children, the family still plays a crucial role in the necessary changes.

The need for them is indisputable. "Without changes in diet and exercise and smoking and the other risk factors," says Albert McClure, a clinical coordinator at Humana, "we've seen bypass surgery patients returning within five years or even two or three years for a second surgery. Then they realize that a bypass isn't going to last unless you take good care of it. Those patients are ready to make changes. I have no trouble motivating them; two surgeries are enough to motivate anybody." But most of the changes are terrifically harder to make if everyone around you continues the old patterns. "The whole family has to commit to lifestyle changes," insists McClure. "And to accomplish that, they have to understand the need for it. That's why it's important for them to be educated along with the patient."

And that, of course, is why this chapter exists.

------

* Lipids are fats. The combining form of the word is "lipo," as in "lipoprotein," which you'll see in "Cholesterol" in chapter 4.

What's Done About It

As a nation, we have become very aware of risk factor modification. Through the evolution of medical science and clinical practice, we can identify causes and circumstances that lead to heart disease, we can spot genetic defects. And there is virtually nothing that affects the heart that cannot be treated today—with medications, bypass surgery, valve replacement, angioplasty, and transplantation.

> —Dr. Jack Matloff
> Director
> Department of Thoracic and
> Cardiac Surgery
> Cedars-Sinai Medical Center
> Los Angeles

Dr. Lawrence Cohn is talking specifically about surgery, but what he says applies to virtually all treatments for all heart conditions:

If there's one thing I would say to families after, say, a successful bypass operation, it's that this is not a curative operation. All these operations are palliative. That is, they make the symptoms better and they increase longevity, but they don't cure the cause of the problem, which is a combination of genetic influences and various controllable risk factors such as diet, smoking, stress, and the others.

An operation can't eradicate the cause, even though the patient is helped a lot. It's not curative. What that means is that patient and family have to attack all the factors that cause the disease process. Diet, exercise, avoidance of stress, better working habits, more sleep—all those kinds of things have to be watched.

A lot of people have the misconception that, "Well, now I've had the bypass, everything's cool, and I don't have to worry about it." They go back to smoking, and other things. And five years later they're back for another operation.

Treatment may eradicate heart disease symptoms, hugely improve the quality of life, make a perfectly normal life possible. Still, the underlying cause of the condition always lurks in the body, always threatens a return. With that understood, though, today's treatments are marvelous.

A Typical Case

For an overview of the possibilities in today's treatment, we asked Dr. Richard J. Gray, director of surgical cardiology at Cedars-Sinai in Los Angeles, to make up a typical case. You'll find unfamiliar terms discussed in the entries below. Dr. Gray asks us to imagine . . .

A 62-year-old man with a history of stable angina pain has been treated successfully with medication for a number of years. Suddenly the pain occurs while the man is at rest, not—as usual—while he's exercising. Rightly alarmed, he calls his cardiologist and meets him immediately at the hospital.

The doctor runs some quick tests, and afterward says to the man, "It looks like you're in the midst of a heart attack."

Reperfusion therapy is indicated, so the patient gets intravenous streptokinase. The pain begins to subside rather suddenly. The EKG shows an improvement. He has a few extra heart beats which are easily controlled with medication. The pain has a sudden increase, then goes away. The EKG returns to some semblance of normal, but with evidence suggesting that a small heart attack has occurred; the blood test shows there is a small amount of heart damage. It's now 6 hours after the pain began.

He stays in the hospital several more days on heparin therapy, then they do an angiogram which shows a very severe blockage in the blood vessel that feeds the area of this small heart attack. The cardiologist sees damage to the heart muscle on the angiogram, but it is relatively small and the rest of the heart seems to move normally.

In addition to this severe blockage—let's say the streptokinase has improved it from complete blockage to 85%—there are blockages between 50 and 75% in the other two major coronary vessels. With all three blocked, angioplasty isn't indicated. But bypass surgery is recommended, especially to prevent the likelihood of a second event in the area that's blocked 85%.

He's operated on, he does well, the story ends happily, and he goes home.

Now, this is a scenario we just didn't see ten years ago: somebody has this heart attack that is arrested in the early minutes, and then we go on to even more definitive therapy to prevent another.

Angiography (Also see "Testing," below)

This key diagnostic test in cardiology merits an entry of its own. Angiography is an extension of cardiac catheterization.* Doctors insert the catheter, a thin, hollow, plastic tube, into an artery, generally in the groin, and carefully, guided by x-ray views all the way, snake it along to the coronary artery (see illustration section following page 16). In cardiac catheterization—a separate test often used to diagnose valve and congenital heart defects—doctors attach the catheter to a gauge to measure pressure in the heart chambers and vessels. In angiography, they pump a dye through the catheter into the coronary arteries. The dye provides contrast for the x-ray movies taken of the heart and its arteries at work. Called "angiograms," these movies are indispensable as the only diagnostic tools that definitively show doctors whether coronary arteries are blocked and how badly, whether there's damage to the heart and how much.

Only two things need concern you about angiography. First, it's relatively expensive, often running around $5,000. More important, you shouldn't let just any "qualified" doctor do it.

Doctors call certain procedures "invasive," from "invade." Whenever you put anything except food and water into the body, especially when you do it by cutting any size hole in the skin, you run some risk. "We will all tell you," says Dr. Simon H. Stertzer, director of medical research at the San Francisco Heart Institute, "that an angiogram can take 10 minutes in the hands of an expert, and has a mortality rate less than one-tenth of 1%, one in a 1000." In fact, one study revealed not a single death among 11,000 random angiograms. Still, major complications, such as damage to the arteries, precipitation of arrhythmia, heart attack, or stroke, do run between 1 and 2%. That risk is small; but why not cut it to the vanishingly tiny? "I wouldn't go to a colleague who does three a week," says Dr. Stertzer; "I'd go to someone who does nothing *but* angiography." Although even routinely competent hands make the risk small, you want an expert.

---

* Originally, "catheter" meant a tube inserted into body cavities to remove fluids—the most familiar use (any way you look at it) being the tube that drains urine after surgery.

Angioplasty*

Doctors work a catheter into the blocked coronary artery (see "Angiography," above), and insert, through the catheter, a smaller one tipped with an uninflated, hotdog-shaped balloon. When they have wedged the balloon into what's left of the opening in the plaque blocking that artery, they inflate the balloon. That compacts the plaque, forcing the arterial opening wider. Guidelines from the American College of Cardiology and the American Heart Association say that to be considered successful, an angioplasty must widen the arterial opening by more than 20%, leave it less than 50% blocked, and decidedly not cause a heart attack or the need for emergency bypass surgery. When successful, angioplasties substitute brilliantly for more expensive, painful, and risky surgery. Doctors across the U.S. performed about 200,000 angioplasties in 1988. Not all succeeded.

Does that mean there were too many? Not enough? Were they performed by the right people? The somewhat complex answers form a body of knowledge you should ponder before anyone performs angioplasty on anyone in your family.

Dr. Lawrence Cohn of Boston, himself a cardiac surgeon, says, "There are many patients for whom angioplasty should be done instead of surgery. It's very good for certain subsets of patients." That subset includes many like the patient Dr. William DeVries saw in Louisville: "A football coach came in, almost dead; he had an angioplasty, and was coaching the game that Saturday—without surgery!" *With* surgery he still would have been in the hospital on Saturday.

But that's not the whole story. Dr. Cohn also says, "I don't see angioplasty as a panacea. I think it's overused." It induces patients who need surgery to delay, hoping that the balloon will save them from the knife. "Obviously I can understand that," Cohn continues. "If they have a situation where a balloon will work, and it does work, great! But that's a fairly small number of people, actually."

And if it doesn't work, disaster can follow. "As you'd expect," explains Dr. Richard Gray, "when you blow this balloon up it totally closes off the blood vessel, usually for 20 or 30 seconds. Sometimes a blood clot forms, completely blocking the artery, and a heart attack may ensue. Some are opened by using the balloon again, or

---

* Also called "balloon angioplasty"; formal name "percutaneous transluminal coronary angioplasty," or PTCA. "Per" = "through," "cutaneous" = "skin," "trans" = "across," and "lumen" = "opening in a tube," in this case the one in coronary arteries through which, if it weren't clogged with plaque, blood would flow (see illustration section following page 16).

by medication that dissolves blood clots. But some people are taken to the operating room as an emergency." The problem remains serious enough so that guidelines insist that a surgical team stand by in the hospital, ready to perform emergency bypass, whenever angioplasty is scheduled.

The head of cardiac anesthesia at a city hospital once accosted Dr. Simon Stertzer, one of the nation's pioneers in angioplasty, and said, "You guys have done us a great disservice: three times a week patients come to open heart surgery in cardiac arrest, with residents pumping on their chests, because of failed angioplasty."

That sort of talk infuriates Dr. Stertzer. The problem is not with angioplasty, he maintains, but with some of those who practice it today. "The angioplasty emergency surgery rate in an average population shouldn't be more than 30 cases in a 1000," he insists. And of those, most should go to surgery with hardware holding the artery open until a bypass can reperfuse the heart muscle. Even if the artery is closed, the patient should reach surgery all right because, except for special circumstances,* Stertzer and other experts perform angioplasty only on patients with general heart performance robust enough to survive the off-chance of a closed vessel. "So even when we go to surgery," says Stertzer, "we're sending the surgeon a reasonably stable patient."

Then why the anesthesiologist's complaint? "Because," says Stertzer, "there is a large element of poor angioplasty being done around the country. There are many cardiologists who are doing angioplasty and accepting a complication rate that is outrageously high." They want the prestige of doing this hot new procedure, yet in fact don't do enough of them to become expert. If three a week are not enough to assure a practiced hand at angiography (see above), three surely are not enough for the greater complexities of angioplasty.

Then how can the emergency surgery rate stay only about 3.5%, with mortality under 1%? Because, in fact, the majority of angioplasties performed are not complex. Even the three-a-week cardiologist manages them perfectly well.

Dr. Stertzer has two quarrels with the whole situation. The first harkens back to Dr. Cohn's opinion that only a relatively small number of cases benefit from angioplasty. Stertzer sees that as honest but wrong. He maintains that even the most eminent surgeons do not realize how complex cases can be—and still be treatable *by an*

---

* Cases so severe that the only alternatives are certain death if nothing is done and probable death in surgery, but with a glimmer of hope from a salvage angioplasty.

angioplasty specialist. They arrive at such opinions because the successful angioplasties they see are almost invariably the straightforward cases, while complex cases too often end up in emergency surgery. "The major advance in the last five years," says Stertzer, "is the sophistication of equipment that permits us to do angioplasty on increasingly large numbers of patients who would otherwise need bypass surgery. I would venture to say that 75% of the surgical candidates can have angioplasty."

Unfortunately, Stertzer asserts, not enough of those who perform angioplasty have access to such equipment or know how or when to use it; they may not even recognize the need for special measures. That's his second quarrel with the general state of the art today: too many doctors do angioplasties beyond their competence. It's all a matter of training and experience.* "We do many here that are failed angioplasties elsewhere," says Stertzer. "It isn't because of the physical dexterity in my ten fingers. It's because I know what to use for some particular problem that has escaped somebody else because they do three a week, which is just not enough for this type of problem."

That does not mean you must automatically rush to San Francisco for angioplasty. Specialists abound throughout the country. Not that you necessarily need one; most cases are simple. The key is confidence. "If you're with a cardiologist who does other things besides angioplasty," says Stertzer, "do you have the confidence that he will know what his limitations are?" If so, that's ideal. Stertzer continues:

> You may find somebody who does those three a week who is honest about his limitations and who sees that *this* is his kind of case: "I know what equipment to use, what the complexity of the problem is; I've been dealing with this kind of problem for eight years; I have good surgical standby; I know I can't do certain things that angioplasty experts can do—but it's ridiculous to send *this* case out because it's so simple."
>
> The same way it would be absurd for a general practitioner to send somebody with a common cold to an infectious disease specialist.

Surely that program makes sense for everyone.

---

* Dr. Andreas Gruntzig developed angioplasty and performed the first in Zurich, Switzerland in 1977. He shared his technique with Dr. Richard Myler in San Francisco and with Dr. Stertzer in New York. At first, angioplasty met with skepticism from the profession. When Stertzer moved west in 1983, he was still the only physician in New York doing angioplasties. He and Myler are now both at the San Francisco Heart Institute, located in Daly City, a suburb. Dr. Gruntzig was killed in a plane crash in 1985.

Arrhythmia

Not all arrhythmias require medical intervention; some involve little danger or discomfort. Others disappear once doctors control their basic cause, such as infections, low potassium, or congestive heart failure. By the same token, when the underlying cause is serious enough—extreme, uncontrollable congestive heart failure, for instance—the arrhythmia is only a symptom of the even more threatening condition, and will reappear even if "controlled" for the moment. Nevertheless, doctors can intervene effectively with many arrhythmias.

The first level of intervention is medication. Some drugs keep irritated parts of the heart from starting contractions; others regulate the heart's usual electrical circuit; still others work directly on the ventricle to slow down or speed up its contractions. Doctors give these drugs intravenously in emergencies, orally for long-term use. "Unfortunately," says Dr. Prediman K. Shah, director of inpatient cardiology and the CCUs of Cedars-Sinai in Los Angeles, "when the heart muscle is extremely weak, the side effects can be more sinister that the original problem: gastrointestinal symptoms, dizziness, lightheadedness. And in some patients, the drugs may actually precipitate a worse arrhythmia." Such patients are obviously very hard to treat.

Another level of treatment is cardioversion, an electric shock strong enough to blank out all electrical activity in the heart for a moment. Cleared of arrhythmic signals, the heart's electrical system can start fresh in the correct pattern. However, unless doctors eliminate the underlying cause of the arrhythmia, it generally reappears: often quite soon, generally in a matter of months.

Defibrillation is emergency cardioversion, specifically for the deadly ventricular fibrillation. Doctors sometimes implant a special defibrillating device in the chests of some patients; it delivers the necessary shock directly to the heart muscle whenever a life-threatening arrhythmia occurs.

When the heart beats too slowly, doctors may implant a pacemaker (see "Hardware," below). One type takes over the heart's normal signal-sending duties, sparking at a preset rate. The other type takes over only when it senses a heart beat lower than some predetermined minimum.

Despite problems that still plague arrhythmia management, note how far medicine has come in dealing with what used to be almost intractable. "We have a greater understanding of why arrhythmias occur and what to do about them," says Dr. Richard Gray. "The situation is a lot better than 10 years ago."

Bypass Surgery*

First performed in the late 1960s, this is now routine surgical treatment to forestall heart attacks that are judged likely to happen by angiography and other tests, and to restore blood flow to areas of the heart damaged by heart attacks. In some instances, surgeons can do bypasses while a heart attack is in progress, saving the affected heart muscle. They now do close to 300,000 bypasses a year in the United States.

"Bypass" describes the operation exactly (see illustration section following page 16). Cardiac surgeons take a section of vein from another part of the patient's body. They split the breast bone† to get at the heart, cut a tiny hole in the patient's aorta, sew one end of the vein over the hole so that blood will flow into the vein, then similarly attach the other end of the vein to a spot below the place where plaque blocks the coronary artery. Blood from the aorta bypasses the obstruction, once again feeding the part of the heart that was getting little or no blood because of the blockage.

Quite often more than one artery is blocked, so surgeons will perform multiple bypasses. Depending on how many they do, and the patient's condition, the operation takes between four and six hours. While the surgical team works directly on the heart, the patient is hooked up to a heart-lung machine, which performs the function of those two organs so that the heart can be at rest. (You can imagine the difficulty doing fine stitchery on a *beating* heart!) Stopping the heart may sound scary, but it is now entirely routine.

Surgeons generally take the bypass vein‡ from the leg; it's one that's not necessary for perfectly adequate circulation. Increasingly, though, instead of a vein, surgeons use one or both of the internal mammary arteries, which supply blood to the chest wall. In that case they leave the upper end of the artery where it is and graft the lower end onto the coronary artery below the blockage.

For some unknown reason mammary arteries seldom accumulate plaque, which too readily blocks vein bypasses. One surgeon pronounces them "better than vein grafts." On the other hand, the operation takes

---

* Full, formal name: "coronary bypass surgery."

† This is the reason patients experience pain after the operation and typically look awful for the first day or so. The wound heals quickly, and the bone knits within a couple of months; but that is a major assault on the body, and the body lets you know it doesn't like it.

‡ It's called the "saphenous" vein, which comes through Latin from an Arabic word that means "vein in the leg."

somewhat longer, and patients experience a little more postoperative discomfort. And, of course, each person has only two mammary arteries, while some need more than two bypasses.

The quality, safety, length of time bypasses last, and the number performed represent some of the more dramatic developments since we wrote *Survive.*

Cardiomyopathy

"The first thing we teach them," said a nurse in a cardiac surgical group at Vanderbilt University Hospital, "is what cardiomyopathy is, and why transplantation is the answer, eventually." That answer is the only glimmer of real hope.

For those sufferers with the kind of cardiomyopathy that enlarges and weakens the left ventricle, doctors prescribe restricted activity to reduce strain on the heart. Medications can temporarily handle some of the symptoms: diuretics to reduce water retention, anti-arrhythmic drugs, blood thinners to cut the risk of clots. But, as one authority baldly puts it, deterioration is progressive "and the majority of patients will die within 4 or 5 years" after symptoms begin.

The story is only marginally cheerier for those with the kind of cardiomyopathy in which the ventricle wall thickens, assuming they have the kind in which a thickened septum restricts blood flow to the aorta. Sometimes surgeons can cut away part of the septum. Otherwise, the treatment is to restrict activity and prescribe medications (beta blockers or calcium channel blockers) that permit greater blood flow.

A variation exists if the heart stiffens. One sufferer described a miserable existence with blackouts, bad reaction to some medications, arrhythmias that needed electric defibrillation, and then a pacemaker— in short, no life at all. Finally, he said, after some extensive tests the doctor "came into my room and said, 'I've got some bad news. Your heart is turning into scar tissue, and we think that you're going to require a heart transplant.'"

In fact, as you'll see in chapter 5, that is not necessarily bad news. It is often, quite literally, a life saver.

Cholesterol

We explained in chapter 3 that a disposition toward heart disease can be inherited; that, of course, remains beyond anyone's control. However, many doctors now think that if you can push the cholesterol level down far enough you can offset even a genetic tendency toward clogged arteries. To understand how you can make it happen, and the terms you hear used nowadays, it helps to know something about the mechanics of cholesterol.

Cholesterol does not dissolve in the blood and must be transported in packets of lipoprotein. Five types exist, but only two of them figure in heart disease: high-density lipoprotein (HDL) and low-density lipoprotein (LDL). You'll hear people call these, respectively, "good" and "bad" cholesterol. HDL carries cholesterol away from the arteries to the liver, which disposes of it. LDL circulates cholesterol throughout the body—usefully to tissue cells, where it forms membranes; destructively to the coronary arteries, where it helps form plaque.

For adults, the most often quoted guidelines suggest a total cholesterol level reading below 200.* From 200 up to 240 is a suspect range. Between 240 and 260, one stands at moderate risk, and above 260 at high risk. Just as important, HDL should constitute at least 25% of one's total cholesterol—the higher the percentage the better. That means the higher the HDL number the better; indeed if it falls below 35, you may be in trouble. Any time the LDL number hits 160 (lower with demonstrated heart disease and two or more major risk factors), you may be in trouble.

On the sunny side, for every 1% you lower your cholesterol, you cut the risk of coronary heart disease by 2%. You offset unfortunate genes with total cholesterol no higher than 180, HDL around 50, and LDL no higher than 130. Dr. Hillel Laks says that if they get patients' readings down to that level, after bypass surgery, "we should be successful in preventing progression of the disease." He goes on to say, "we know that people who have these very low cholesterols tend rarely to get coronary artery disease."

The first step is knowing where you are, and "you" means everyone in the family, the patient, yourself, the children (figures for them are different; ask a doctor). Of course you want to be sure the test results are accurate and standard each time, especially since cholesterol levels vary naturally with such elements as stress. Kevan Shaheen, nurse manager of the Lipid Center at Humana in Louisville suggests:

> Always get the testing done at the same lab, and ask them or your doctor what your numbers are—don't be satisfied with "They're OK." You need to know what the numbers are and keep records of them so

---

* What's being measured is the amount of cholesterol in a certain amount of blood; the terms used are milligrams and deciliters. Neither term means anything to most of us, which scarcely matters so long as the measuring unit stays constant and we all measure the same thing all the time.

you're aware of where you're going. It helps to make long-term change if you're aware the changes you're making are doing something for you. Make a comparison after you've done your diet work for 6 weeks and 3 months and so on.

Shaheen also advises that you make sure the lab does the same things the same way each time. They should instruct you not to eat and drink for about 12 hours before the test; they should have you sit still or lie down for about 5 minutes before blood is drawn.

How do you make cholesterol levels sink? Your main weapon is diet. You want to reduce the amount of cholesterol eaten; more important, you want to reduce the total amount of fat eaten, especially the animal fats and polysaturated vegetable fats (for details see chapter 10). The only possible exceptions to that are fatty fish and shellfish; their fatty acids (Omega-3) tend to increase HDL.* So does exercise. On the other end of the seesaw, oat bran may help reduce the blood's LDL, although you must eat a forbidding amount of the stuff to do much good.

Fads absolutely teem in this field. As we write this, a book extolling the glories of oat bran is a best-seller. The fact is, miracles in the field do not occur. Sensible, steady diet does the job, and the get-thin-quick and cut-cholesterol-quick schemes have just about as much merit as the get-rich-quick ones.

How about pills? Experts at a recent American Medical Association symposium agreed that the number of people who need drug therapy to lower cholesterol is somewhere between 1 and 8% of the whole population; that is, those with a severe genetic predisposition to high cholesterol. If anyone in your family needs drugs such as lovastatin and niacin, a doctor must be involved, and the side effects can be unpleasant. Correct diet is a *much* preferable way to lower cholesterol.

Clot Dissolvers† (Streptokinase and TPA)
(Also see "Medication," below)

When a blood clot forms, completely shutting a narrowed coronary artery, the part of the heart fed by that artery starts to die. But its death is neither sudden nor rapid. "If you can restore blood flow before all the heart muscle is dead," explains one doctor, "you can abort whatever remaining damage would have been done." The way to do that is to dissolve the clot that's blocking the blood flow—and

---

* You can't eat HDL, but things you eat can encourage the body to produce more.

† Doctors call them "thrombolytics," from two Greek words meaning . . . guess what?

this "thrombolytic therapy" is what the same doctor calls "the real revolution in heart attack management." He is Dr. Sam Teichman, director of professional services at Genentech, the genetic engineering bio-pharmaceutical company that produces TPA, newest clot dissolver on the market.* Naturally, he's biased. But Dr. Eugene Braunwald agrees, and he has no ax to grind. He's chairman of Harvard's department of medicine, physician-in-chief at Boston's Brigham & Women's Hospital. He said, "it's a very exciting time," as he contemplated a new study that showed TPA treatment slashing the death rate from heart attacks.

Although researchers find that a clot dissolver seems to do some good if administered as much as 24 hours after a heart attack, the most effective time to start the therapy is within four hours. Doctors introduce a clot dissolver into the bloodstream intravenously, or by catheter directly into the artery. Either way, it quickly destroys the clot and allows blood to flow through the (to be sure, still narrowed) artery. Dr. Zahi H. Masri, surgeon at Humana in Louisville, says, "We've had many cases where a patient treated with streptokinase either ended up with a smaller heart attack, where the heart muscle was still viable, or you saved that area completely. In either case you buy time to allow you to do other things: balloon angioplasty or bypass surgery or whatever the patient needs."

Another study among 17,000 patients showed that a combination of streptokinase and aspirin cut the death rate by another 50%.

What's the difference between streptokinase and TPA? Effectiveness and side effects, probably; certainly about $2,000 a dose. Streptococcal bacteria produce streptokinase, so allergic reactions can produce problems. And if the patient ever had a strep throat, the body has built up a resistance that can blunt streptokinase's action.

The initials "TPA" stand for "tissue plasminogen activator," the body's own clot dissolving agent, a protein that Genentech scientists purified, analyzed, and now can synthesize in quantity. "TPA represents an advantage over streptokinase," says Genentech's Dr. Teichman. "It's human protein rather than bacterial, so allergic reactions and resistance present no problems. Recombinant DNA technology used to make TPA allows greater purity. TPA proves more potent, both in test tube and in patients; dose for dose, more clot dissolving ability."

It also costs over 10 times more: a dose of streptokinase runs about $200; the price of a dose of TPA is $2,200. In early 1988, the

---

* Apsac, described as "a super-duper streptokinase," is still being tested and is not yet on the market.

government boggled at the price, compared with the added advantages of TPA, and refused supplemental Medicare payments for the treatment—a decision Harvard's Dr. Braunwald promptly denounced.

The only negative for both treatments is some tendency to cause bleeding, which Dr. Teichman says is rarely a real danger; more a matter of doctors' wary perception. In any case, clot dissolving treatment represents a revolution in heart attack management.

Heart Attack (Myocardial Infarction)

It's so heartening, let's repeat what we quoted before:

The treatment for heart attack is never just "Go to bed for six weeks" any more. We're out of that realm completely; we're into a totally activist approach—the combination of thrombolytic agents, balloons, surgery, and all this. It is saving lives, no question.

—Dr. Lawrence Cohn

Just as important, this activist approach lengthens the lives it saves and markedly improves their quality.

You can see the details under the separate entries, "Clot Dissolvers," "Angioplasty," and "Bypass," and get a feeling for the sweep of what today's cardiologists do by looking at "A Typical Case" at the start of this chapter. Briefly, depending on how soon they catch the patient after the heart attack starts, doctors use sophisticated tests to pinpoint where a clot has blocked an artery; then they can prevent any damage to the heart muscle or, at least, minimize the amount of damage by administering clot dissolvers that let blood once again flow through the artery. Next, they can either widen the narrowed artery with angioplasty or surgically bypass the narrowed spot. Either way, they enormously reduce chances of another heart attack.

Finally, ideally, the patient enters a rehabilitation program (see chapter 11) to build up the body, along with the heart, lungs, and circulatory system, and to start a lifestyle calculated to lower risk of further heart disease.

Not everyone qualifies for such treatment. Age, condition, the mildness or severity of the attack, the number of arteries affected, the time elapsed before reaching a hospital—even the sophistication of equipment and personnel at the hospital—these and other circumstances may rule out some or all new interventions. No matter. Today, activism touches even "traditional" treatment.

As in the old days, doctors and nurses immediately calm the patient and alleviate the pain, two essentials for reducing strain on the heart. But today's pain killers are more effective; and calming is more credible since, today, the medical team can *do* something about the attack. Thanks to sensitive tests and monitoring devices, they safely start patients on rehabilitative exercise within a few days—walking and aerobic exercises that raise the heart rate to levels that are strengthening yet safe.

At the same time, medications are more effective today, and they exist in such profusion that the right combination for each patient is easier to find.

In two weeks or less, many patients are home, soon afterward embarked on a formal, long-term rehab program that is so effective, it can even make it possible for those with uncorrectable angina to be active in ways that, before, would have left them clutching their chests and fumbling for nitro tablets.

Hardware (Also see "Technology, Future," below)

Some of the doctor's weapons against heart disease are devices that help treat various conditions or simply buy time until treatment is possible.

Swan-Ganz Catheter

Starting in 1970, this device provided doctors with a revolutionary system for monitoring conditions from *within* the heart. It let them analyze exactly the effect of medications and other aspects of coronary care.

"Now," says Dr. William Ganz, co-developer of the device, "even a physician without special training can insert this *flexible* catheter at the patient's bedside to accurately measure pressures from within the vessels and the heart. They no longer have to move the patient to a special x-ray unit for the lengthy procedure of inserting a stiff catheter."

Pacemaker

Battery-driven, and implanted in the chest of a patient with severe arrhythmia problems, it takes the place of the body's natural pacemaker (the sinus node), sending regular signals that restore measured rhythm to the contractions of the atria and ventricles.

*Intraaortic Balloon Pump**

An IABP can keep a very weak heart beating, and out of cardiac shock, until doctors can do something definitive. They insert the

---

* This is entirely different from balloon angioplasty.

balloon into the aorta. Inflating and deflating with the heart beat, the pump helps push blood through the aorta and out of the heart, making the heart's job easier. At the same time, it forces more blood into the coronary arteries, better feeding the heart muscle.

Left Ventricular Assist Device

A surgeon implants an LVAD, weighing 1.5 pounds, about the size of a fist, next to the heart. One tube brings blood into it from the left ventricle; another tube runs blood from the LVAD to the aorta. Inside, two concentric pusher plates move alternately toward and away from each other about a centimeter's distance—enough to keep the body's entire blood supply circulating. The LVAD can take some of the burden from a weakened heart or take over the heart's whole job.

Although the LVAD is a boon for the small percentage of patients whose hearts need time to start beating strongly enough on their own, after surgery, and for some in cardiogenic shock after a heart attack, it's used mostly, as Dr. Prediman Shah puts it, "as a bridge to bail patients out of impending doom until a more definitive treatment, such as a transplant, can be performed. It allows people to live through a crisis. In that sense, the LVAD is a very temporizing intervention." For one thing, even with the Novacor LVAD, the only otherwise implantable version, a wire protrudes through the skin to the power supply. However, Dr. William Frist, one of the principal investigators for the Novacor LVAD says, "The prototype for a totally implanted device, including power supply, has been developed and tested in animals, and appears to be very good. At that point nothing will protrude through the skin."

Notice, that's still not an artificial heart: the other three chambers and the valves of a heart helped by an LVAD must still function. But it comes close, and brings us to:

The Artificial Heart

We discuss this more fully below in "Technology, Future" because, as one doctor regretfully says, "right now, with the artificial heart, I think it's back to the drawing board to study more about its problems and its intricacies."

Publicity has certainly ventilated its problems; there have been no long-term survivors. But overlooked in the noise has been the fact that artificial hearts demonstrably *work;* they do keep people alive long enough to receive successful transplants.

Medication

The drugs that doctors prescribe today are diverse, sophisticated, with a function and potency nicely calibrated to the patient's need; they are very effective. The most impressive testimonial to their effectiveness, oddly enough, is the fact that today's surgeons perform more bypasses as emergencies, with the patient in heart attack or with unstable angina, than as elective surgeries where there's still plenty of time. It's because symptoms and conditions that doctors once could control only with surgery now yield to various medications for so long that when the medications finally fail, the condition has progressed to emergency proportions.

Everyone in the family should know what drugs the patient needs and why*: what the drugs do, what the side effects may be, what the signs are that something (like the dosage) needs adjustment. That way, everyone will be alert to the need for the patient's faithfully taking the prescribed drugs and for monitoring reactions. The prescribing doctor will almost surely explain; if you forget, or need further clarification, the pharmacist who fills the prescription can help.

The assortment of medications available today is marvelous. Nitrates (such as nitroglycerin) widen arteries; calcium channel blockers prevent them from narrowing in spasms. Beta blockers slow the heart and make it contract less vigorously so it requires less blood; digitalis makes it pump harder. Other drugs reduce high blood pressure, thin the blood, keep blood clots from forming, rid the body of excess salt and water, control arrhythmias, and lower cholesterol. Dr. Emmanuel Horovitz's book, *Heart Beat* (see page 112), gives a clear, cogent rundown with comprehensive descriptions.

A word about generic drugs. If you can read the handwriting, you'll note that a doctor usually specifies drugs by brand name. A pharmacist may offer you a generic substitute—the same drug or mixture under its chemical name—because, while the generic costs you less, the pharmacist makes a greater profit margin. It may not be a good buy. The doctor knows the quality of the brand name and trusts it; who knows about the generic? Dr. Leon Resnekov says,

> The generic may be a good and reliable product. The problem is that the patient and the physician have no way to know. We have no idea where the pharmacist buys it, who the manufacturer is. Some generic drugs have been very poor productions, including some that the

---

* It's a good idea to write them down, carrying one list in wallet or purse, taping another inside the bathroom medicine cabinet.

hospital, here, has bought. We may be the University of Chicago Medical Center, but the head of our pharmacy has to cut costs, too, so he buys some generic drugs. Well, some of those drugs have been absolutely hopeless.

Your best strategy, if offered a sizable generic saving, is to check with your doctor.

We end on the happy note that one "medication" is a moderate amount of alcohol, no more than two drinks a day, wine, beer or spirits. In fact, for some unclear reason, non-drinkers run a higher risk of heart disease than such moderate drinkers do.

Smoking

Motivation for you and the rest of the family to stop smoking should be obvious. If you smoke, it makes quitting all the harder for the patient. And the patient *must* quit. It's no longer a matter of "someday smoking will catch up with you." As we explained in chapter 3, for anyone with heart disease smoking can be instantly fatal.

One former patient we talked with articulates the only sensible attitude. Doctors caught his condition in time to order a bypass before a heart attack struck. As he walked up the steps to the hospital, he says,

> I threw away my last cigarette, and I knew it *was* my last. The doctor had said, "Forget about lung cancer; with your heart disease, you keep smoking and you won't live long enough to get it." You just say to yourself, *not* "I'm going to quit smoking," but "I am *now* a nonsmoker." There's no use worrying about how badly I want a cigarette because I can't have one.

Stress

Many books instruct us in handling stress. The best quick lesson we've seen is a 16-page pamphlet, "A Guide To Managing Stress," available from Krames Communications, 312 90th Street, Daly City, CA 94015.

Most authorities agree that the first step is recognizing when you are under stress, then changing whatever elements you can that cause the stress. You learn to walk away from certain situations and people.

Some you can't avoid. Then, says Dr. Harvey Alpern, "If people can interject periods of relaxation into their lives and take the stress off themselves on a regular basis, even if they can't do anything else about the stress, that helps." He suggests practicing relaxation therapy for 10 or 15 minutes once or twice a day; you can learn the technique easily from a book, *The Relaxation Response,* by Dr. Herbert Benson and Miriam Z. Klipper.

Professionals offer guidance in similar relaxation techniques, plus variations like biofeedback and guided imagery. Most rehabilitation programs cover stress (see chapter 11).

Another important element: make vacations truly relaxing—not hectic scrambles, with the whole family, plus maybe pets, crammed into the car for a 10-day, 2,000 mile trek. "The ideal," says Dr. Alpern, "is a three-day holiday, perhaps even once a month, fairly close by with just spouse or other relevant individual (or by yourself) doing something you find really relaxing."

If all else fails, a few patients need formal psychological counseling, generally available through hospital referral services.

Families commonly make the mistake of reflexively urging their patient to stop work (if that's financially possible) under the misapprehension that not working automatically solves the stress problem. Far from it. "Spouses ask me, 'Should he go back to work?'" says Dr. Frederick Grover. "And I say, 'Does he enjoy his work?' If so, then by all means he should go back to work because otherwise he'll go nuts. Now, if he can't stand his job, if it makes him nervous and upset, then sure, it's good therapy to stop, if possible, or change." Of course "he" and "she" are interchangeable.

The family's proper role goes far beyond the negative of not discouraging a return to work. Indeed that role is so important that Laura Cupper, vocational rehab counselor in Ottawa, says, "I prefer a patient's family to be an integral part of the decision-making process about a patient's work, and to hear all the discussions first hand."

Technology, Future

If we look where we've been, and look to where we're going, the horizon is really unlimited.

—Dr. William DeVries
Artificial heart pioneer

The advances that brought us to today's Aggressive Age of heart disease management continue. But doctors urge two cautions. "Often we have to counsel patients and their families about 'the magic bullet' syndrome," says Dr. William Dafoe; "they neglect their health, hoping for some magical cure." No one is even working on a "cure" for heart disease; awe-inspiring as promised technology is, it remains palliative, not curative.

The second caution is treated below in "Your Role." No one is working on a substitute for tender loving care, either: that's your department.

Otherwise, the future's rosy.

Start at the small end with what's often overlooked. "The longer your experience with any technique," says Dr. Warren Goldburgh, "the more apt you are to evolve better applications and better indications for restraint." For instance, reperfusion therapy represented a major breakthrough: clot dissolvers, angioplasty, and bypass now flood threatened heart muscle with life-giving blood. Dr. Sam Teichman says, "It's hard to see where the next major breakthrough will come in this field." Instead, he looks for advances in knowledge of how *best* to reperfuse the heart.

For transplants (see chapter 5), the outlook continues even brighter. Dr. Leon Resnekov expects giant strides in techniques "to damp down the rejection process," the body's persistent attempt to eliminate alien tissue. "The future looks much better than any of us would have predicted years ago. What's truly amazing is the speed at which you can go from basic laboratory work at the sophisticated cellular level into the clinical arena with new knowledge that's directly applicable to a patient."

Dr. William Frist predicts, "we'll have a *good* artificial heart" within seven or eight years, one that approximates the success rate doctors now expect from human heart transplants. Dr. William DeVries, the first surgeon to implant an artificial heart, isn't sure of the timing, but is certain we *shall* have a long-term artificial heart— one so good it will function indistinguishably from a healthy organ— "because there's a great need for it; it can help people, and society demands it."

Many new techniques associated with angioplasty now receive much attention and generate considerable excitement—maybe too much, and certainly prematurely, according to Dr. Stertzer, who helped pioneer angioplasty and still leads in experimentation with the new techniques.

Lasers, for example, can burn a hole into plaque, allowing doctors to wedge a balloon catheter into arteries that, before, resisted angio- plasty. Doctors also use lasers to heat a metal "hot tip," which burns the required hole in the plaque. Other cold (excimer) lasers destroy plaque with high-energy waves in ways that may not even require angioplasty afterwards. Doctors are also testing atherectomy—catheters that pare away, suction, or gouge out plaque. Once doctors reopen an artery, they can now insert various mechanical devices, called "stents," to keep them open—like shoring up the sides of a tunnel.

Unfortunately, Dr. Stertzer warns, all these *are* still experimental. He fears that "hype," especially about space-age–sounding lasers, may distort the research process and divert attention from more productive, if less newsworthy, advances in basic technique. Lasers and hot tips, he says, have proved themselves in clearing arteries of the leg, where the channel is straight, repair surgery is easy if something goes wrong, and where, anyway, the patient's life is not at stake. Using lasers in the narrow, twisting coronary arteries—where perforation of the wall (or other damage) could be fatal—that is another matter. "The laser does not yet have a defined role in the heart," says Dr. Stertzer. "It may in the next four or five years, and I'm going to get a lot more information in the next two years."

The same thing applies to stents: by 1991 doctors should have a firmer idea about their value and best use. Meanwhile, Dr. Stertzer sees atherectomy—the Roto-rooter principle—as the most likely new field for investigation. But, he says, the best news in angioplasty is still the increasing sophistication of basic equipment that allows experts to treat ever greater numbers of patients. That process continues.

So does development of miniature pumps that, like the LVAD, take over part or all of the heart's work, letting it rest and heal. A new one, the Hemopump, is tiny enough, $\frac{1}{4}$ inch wide and $\frac{1}{2}$ inch long— about the size of a pencil eraser—to operate inside the left ventricle.

Canadian researches are developing a balloon catheter that can map diseased areas of the ventricle, the ones causing arrhythmias, then destroy them with an electric shock.

The most encouraging thing about technology today is the fact that by the time you read this, new wonders will likely be well on the way to making some of what we've discussed obsolete.

Testing

Dr. Simon Stertzer, an expert in angiography, says that "the greatest thing to hit this country in the evaluation of heart disease in middle aged people is the ability to do it *without* an invasive procedure like angiography." No matter how quick and safe angiography is in expert hands, it does require insertion of a catheter into the heart. A number of tests that, at worst, call for only a hypodermic needle are now of stunning sophistication and accuracy. The one that Dr. Stertzer specifically had in mind is called the "stress-thallium" test. While the patient walks on a motor-driven treadmill (stress test), doctors inject a small, safe amount of radioactive thallium-201 into the bloodstream. The heart's muscle cells that are being perfused by blood in a normal way absorb the thallium; dead tissue and tissue being starved of blood do not. After exercise, the pattern of absorption shows up on a scintillation camera. Any part of the heart not getting the blood it needs announces itself because of its lack of thallium. A repeat scan some hours later tells the doctor if the lack of blood is temporary or permanent. It is remarkably accurate. Dr. Stertzer says,

> When I hit age 45 I decided I would do a stress-thallium. If that was negative, I'd be satisfied. It doesn't guarantee that the arteries are entirely normal, but it does tell me that there's no highgrade obstruction, and therefore no danger of a heart attack within, say, 18 months.
>
> Now, that's unprecedented: that we are able to determine with some certainty—without going inside the body—that a person of 45 or 55 or whatever age is *not* liable to have a heart attack within a certain period of time.

Other diagnostic tests impress us only marginally less; they include some that have been around for some time, but are now of much greater accuracy and usefulness, such as the familiar EKG (electrocardiogram), which measures the small electrical discharges of the heart during its beating cycle. Changes, especially during exercise, alert the doctor to the probability of heart disease. So doctors often combine an EKG with a treadmill or stationary bicycle stress test.

To get a long-range reading of arrhythmias, they can use a "Holter* EKG," a portable recorder patients wear 24 hours while going through their daily routines (including sex, if they're so inclined).

Echocardiography, in various versions, uses sound waves to display the heart's structure and motion, and speed of the blood within the heart chambers.

Another nuclear scanning test, the "blood pool scan," shows how the ventricle is beating. The "wall motion" part of this test is what one doctor calls "a poor man's angiogram."

"But why," some may wonder, "settle for less when angiography is the definitive test—and will almost surely be performed, anyway, if other tests are positive or equivocal?" Because they've become so good they very adequately substitute, in those who need only routine checkups, or in whom heart disease is only a suspicion, for the more expensive, and—no matter how statistically safe—riskier procedure.

---

* This is not a misspelling of "halter," although the recorder is often worn in one; "Holter" is the inventor's name.

Transplants

This is such a new, exciting, and promising field, it deserves its own chapter. See chapter 5.

Valves

For patients with no important or disabling symptoms, the only treatment for many years may be avoidance of heart-straining activity, plus some simple medications, like diuretics to eliminate fluids that make the heart work harder and digitalis for improved pumping.

When faulty valves start to worsen, though, they usually degenerate quickly; the trick is to replace valves that need replacing before the heart sustains irreversible damage.

Although somewhat riskier than bypass surgery, the valve-replacement operation is now routine. The choice is between mechanical valves and biologic valves. Mechanical ones used to be made of plastic and steel in a "ball-in-the-cage" design; newer ones feature discs or leaflets—doors that allow only one-way blood flow—made of a durable carbon. Biologic valves were once all constructed of tissue taken from pigs because it so resembles human tissue that the body does not reject it. They were called "porcine valves." Nowadays researchers also experiment with "bovine pericardial tissue," taken from cows. Mechanical valves last longer (up to 25 years, versus 10–14 years for biologic), but tend to form blood clots, necessitating continued doses of blood thinner. So the choice hinges on such factors as age, tolerance of blood thinners, susceptibility to bleeding, even the likelihood of pregnancy.

Surgical valve repair, rather than replacement, is more rare—once almost always confined to rheumatic fever cases, although new techniques make it suitable for some problems like leaky mitral valves. In addition, a form of angioplasty called "valvuloplasty" can widen some valves that do not fully open.*

Your Role (TLC)

Fifteen years ago, in our first book, we quoted a doctor who said this about hospitals:

---

* As we write this, the Federal Drug Administration has approved valvuloplasty for only one of the four valves, the pulmonary valve. But according to an update to the third edition of Dr. Braunwald's textbook, *Heart Disease*, a work of almost biblical authority, experimentation goes apace with the other valves.

They're a tradeoff. On the plus side, they offer fine medical care, sophisticated machines, and concentrations of well-trained people who know what to do in an emergency and who have all the equipment and medication they need, right at hand.

And it's still a tradeoff.

Because on the minus side, you give up personal warmth and feeling of personal worth. . . . Instead you can feel like an object, a laboratory specimen, something that's being acted on and is strictly replaceable by any other object.

I guess the ideal would be if someone could invent a cardiac monitor that loves you.

Not—we commented at the time—that he values modern medical machines and medications less, he just values love more. And that means you. All of you: spouse, family, everyone who cares about the patient in ways no doctor or nurse, no outsider, however dedicated, can.

In the past 15 years, they have turned those machines and medications, comparatively speaking, into miracles of healing. Have they done *anything* to infuse them with love for the ailing person you love? Quite the contrary. The very marvel of today's technology tends to distance medical people even further from patients. Dr. William DeVries, who otherwise admires technology, finds the trend worrisome.

With the heavy monitoring—machines replacing human functions, computerization of diagnoses—you get into a tremendous problem: depersonalization of patients. They're in a room alone, surrounded by machines; doctors and nurses come in and look at the machines, not the patient. The machines become a barrier between the health care profession and the patient. That's the number one problem advanced technology leads to.

It's a problem only you and your family can solve. If you go about it the right way (see especially chapters 5 and 6), for all the marvels of technology doctors now command, and the even greater ones they will command in the future, you remain one of their strongest weapons in the fight to make your patient's recovery as quick and complete as can be.

We've moved the frontier so far that it is now the social and economic factors that are becoming more important; 11% of our Gross National Product goes into medical care, and the national debate now is over where health care is going. Is there, should there be a limit? These are ethical and moral decisions, and they don't necessarily involve right or wrong medical answers.

Whether or not we, as a society, have the will, interest, and the financial resources to follow through remains the biggest question.

—Dr. Jack Matloff

Transplants

I used to tell them this is still experimental—but no more.

—Dr. Roland Girardet
Transplant Surgeon, Humana

Candidates

Dr. William Frist had just seen the test results. Now he had to break the news.

"He's got a huge heart," he explained to Mrs. P, wife of a new patient at Vanderbilt, a case of severe cardiomyopathy, "and the heart doesn't work. That's why he feels terrible and he doesn't look strong. He's always weak. . . ." His heart pumped only half the amount of blood it should. He could not survive without a heart transplant. "If we wait much longer his lungs will be irreversibly damaged."

The couple understood the need for a transplant. When would it be? Dr. Frist couldn't tell them. "We have problems getting donors," he said. "We don't have more problems than anywhere else, but our problem is bad. It could be anywhere from a week or two weeks to as long as six months or a year. . . ."

"Does he have that much time?" asked Mrs. P.

"I can't tell you that. But," he said, turning to Mr. P, "without the transplant, the odds of your living a year from now are 50%. . . ."

Actually those weren't bad odds; but they suggested urgency in getting Mr. P on the computer list of those waiting for a suitable heart. "I know you sure feel that way," said Dr. Frist. "I sure do," said Mr. P.

There you have the three central themes when a transplant team evaluates candidates.

First, it must be someone who either cannot live, or will not have a life worth living, without a new heart, someone otherwise healthy, with no other life-threatening conditions, and young enough (65 is the usual cutoff point, below 55 preferred) to assure a reasonable life expectancy with the new heart.

Second, it must be someone that the team social worker or psychologist determines will receive enough moral support to see him or her through the ordeal of waiting for a heart, and then through the rigors of post-surgery. (In this case, evidence of support was a wife palpably interested in the patient's welfare.) Examination of the patient's home circumstances tends to be tediously exhaustive because this part of the evaluation process is so crucial. As Barbara Schulman, R.N., C.P.T.C., senior coordinator for the Regional Organ Procurement Agency of Southern California, explains, "In addition to countless medical worries, there are many others: who will cover the cost of surgery, recovery, and the high, ongoing cost of medication? Medicare? private insurance? some combination of agencies? Have any dental problems gone unattended? That could be dangerous after surgery because the anti-rejection medications make any infection a serious concern. There are just so many things to think about and take care of, a patient almost *must* have an environment of active, caring support."

The third theme is the reason for such extreme choosiness about which candidates will get on the list: the acute and chronic lack of hearts. One doctor estimates that somewhere between 20,000 and 30,000 people need a transplant. Two other doctors put it at 15,000. Another thinks it may be "only" 10,000. In any case they mean "per year" because those who don't get a new heart generally die. By 1988, after the number of transplants had risen each year since 1981, the total leveled off at about 1650. No more hearts were available.

For the implications, see "Commitment" and "Family, Role of the" below.

Commitment

"Transplantation," says Dr. William Frist, "is a lifetime commitment."

Patients must understand, says Dr. Roland Girardet, "they will be linked with doctors and hospitals forever."

It works both ways.

Dr. Frist counts the ways:

The operation is just the start. The patient's commitment involves weekly visits for several months, then monthly visits for the rest of the patient's life. It involves periodic surveillance heart biopsies, which are invasive procedures; it involves compliance on the patient's part, where if he doesn't take his pills three times a day he's going to die.*

But, equally, the doctor commits to continuing care and constant availability. The patient must realize that fact, says Dr. Frist, and adjust to the reasons for it:

He has to give me feedback constantly. If he has a low-grade temperature, he doesn't just "shake it off"; he picks up the phone and calls me. And he needs to do that without feeling, "Oh, he's so busy—I don't want to bother him." If we leave patients with a feeling they're bothering us, statistically a percentage of those patients will die.

A simple low-grade temperature may be warning of rejection or infection or some other derangement that the doctor must handle *now.*

Doctors will not approve transplantation for a patient without that willing commitment. Dr. Girardet explains:

There's no point in transplanting someone who will not be willing to come for checkups, or will not take medication as prescribed. He will die; and we don't have hearts we can take off the shelf. The heart is a very rare commodity and we want to be sure we put it in somebody who can use it, and not waste it.

Condition of the Patient

A nurse who deals mostly with transplant recipients says that one concept patients find hard to grasp is why they should be *so* sick— "Why they can't breathe, why they can't walk, why they can't chew *cereal!*"—when everything else, besides their heart, is normal. Of course, with not enough blood being pumped, the entire body, starved for oxygen, deteriorates. As patients grow weaker, their muscles atrophy, rendering them weaker still.

---

* During the first year after transplant, "patients need to take 12 to 25 doses of medicine daily and submit to 15 to 25 biopsies," according to Dr. Lynne W. Stevenson, part of the transplant group at UCLA, in the November 1988 issue of *The Western Journal of Medicine*, p. 572.

A companion puzzle, says someone who had a transplant over three years ago and now regularly visits patients who are waiting for hearts, is this: "most cannot believe that, bad as they feel now, they can *ever* feel good again." But that's the point of restricting transplants to those whose only serious physical problem is an impaired heart. Once the flow of blood is restored, the body can again function normally. It's not automatic; see "Recovery, Long-term" below and chapter 13, "Rehabilitation." The body can, though, recover its normal strength with reasonable rapidity.

One medical group worried that their first transplant recipient was age 56, a grandmother. They wanted the first to go exceptionally well. Would she do all right? Be strong enough? Get back on her feet? She turned out to be their showcase patient, with a rapid, complication-free recovery: "smoothest one we've ever done," says a doctor involved.

Another patient, a young athlete in his 20s, celebrated the fifth anniversary of his transplant by riding a bicycle across the country.

On a personal note, just before his transplant, Arthur Schoenberg, Jane's husband, did not have enough strength to brush his teeth. As we write this, he is, at age 69, back at work and now *walking* the golf course.

Donors

The single most important fact about donors is that there aren't enough for the demand.

Dr. Christiaan Barnard performed the first human heart transplant in 1967. His patient lived 18 days. Unhappily, the body's immune system rejects alien tissue. Barnard and other doctors around the world persevered nevertheless, performing 101 transplants the next year. The survival rate remained so low, however, that the operation became more of an experimental curiosity, with only about 20, total, in the following years until 1981, when doctors at Stanford, under Norman Shumway, began the heart-transplant use of cyclosporine, a drug that suppresses the rejection process.

"Since 1981," says Dr. Frist, "we've seen exponential growth until 1988. Now it's very clear that the curve is flattening off at about 1650 transplants. Why? Because we're donor limited." He cites the need for education: getting doctors to ask for donations, making the public aware of the need to donate. One of his nurses finds the situation so poignant that if she thought she could persuade people, she says, "I'd be willing to do a lot of community work on my own time just to get people aware." Dr. Paul Terasaki, who heads the UCLA Tissue

Typing Laboratory, proposes a plan that would encourage transplant recipients to join in the educational effort.

Education is critical because being "donor limited" is built into the situation. Hearts must come from otherwise healthy people who have suffered an accident or some illness that has rendered them "brain dead" without affecting their hearts or other usable organs. The upper age limit for donors is usually 40, and their hearts must be free from heart disease.

Obviously, this describes few people. Add the fact that, in almost the same breath as the death announcement, someone must ask the grieving next of kin for the donation (or for permission even if the victim had already signed a donor form), and you know why donors are scarce. Forty-four states require that someone ask the families of potential donors for usable organs—heart, lungs, livers, kidneys, corneas, etc. Almost all state driver's licenses have donor forms on the reverse side. The National Kidney Foundation, 30 E. 33rd Street, 11th Floor, Dept. AL, New York, NY 10016, will send anyone complete information on request.

The wife of one bypass patient says about organ donation, "If you can't live, somebody else can. And what a wonderful way of continuing yourself. If somebody else can use my eyes or my heart or my kidneys or my liver, why not give it to the living? Allow somebody else to live." That seems a commendable, inspiring attitude. Nonetheless, questions do disturb some individuals.

Recipients and their families also have questions. Most are treated below in "Questions, 'Stupid.'" The chief remaining question concerns relationship with the donor's family. No formal one exists; neither side knows the other's identity. But how does the donor's family *feel* about it? That must impact recipients' and their family's feelings about being able to continue life only as a result of someone else's death.

Through a chain of unusual circumstances and coincidences, one young recipient in Tennessee met the donor's parents. "Jim felt as though he had always known them, and they felt the same," says the recipient's wife. "They call Jim's son their grandson. We phone all the time and exchange visits. It's always been a measure of comfort for their loss." Then something happened. After 10 years the transplanted heart developed problems; Jim, now in his mid-30s, needed another transplant. "It upset Jim losing Gary's heart mostly because of them: that was all they had left of Gary. But they told him they understood. If it was for his best to lose it, that's what they wanted him to do. And he should still feel part of the family, because that's how they'd feel."

Family, Role of the

> The success of heart transplantation is not only dependent on the surgery and the medications that follow. It is also critically linked to positive feedback and support from the family. I think that's the single most important social factor that contributes to the success of transplants and restoration of quality of life for patients. No question about that. Absolutely!
>
> —Dr. Prediman Shah

Start with what we mentioned above: a caring family may be the deciding factor in a patient's admission to a transplant program. Unless the transplant team sees promise of strong family support, they hesitate to recommend a transplant.* We quoted a doctor; here it is from the other side, the husband of a recipient: "The social workers before the transplant wanted to know what kind of support group Irene would have, who was going to be here to help. It's like, 'What's the use of wasting a heart on you if you have no one to keep you alive after.'"

"I'll tell you," says one recipient, "it's really harder on the family than the patient." Maybe so; but what recipients regularly declare they need and appreciate most from their families requires little: "just to *be* there for you," says a woman waiting for a heart. "I can't say enough about just being there when you need them. And knowing they're just a phone call away." Often it means literally *just* being there. The wife of a patient who, the week before, had died waiting for a suitable transplant says, "You can't give them enough support— and love. Even if you don't say anything. A lot of times, John'd be watching a TV program, and he'd say, "C'mere and sit down. Now, don't say nothing, just sit down." And we'd sit there for hours, and he was content. I'd just be there."

Can the family assume the candidate will take their willingness to be there for granted. "No," says a woman who, three months before, had received a heart/lung transplant. "That needs saying. You need to hear it. Because at that time you're just not sure of anything, and you need to know that there are people out there who love you and will support you and be with you."

We examine other specific parts of the transplant family's role throughout the rest of this chapter.

---

* It's not absolute. "The existence of strong family support is important for compliance and outcome but in most programs is no longer essential for acceptance."—Dr. Lynne Stevenson, quoted in footnote on page 52.

Hardest Part, The

> I've known enough people waiting on transplants that it's *agonizing:* that's probably the hardest part of all of this—the day-to-day thing that Betty's living through right now: you know, tomorrow . . . *maybe.*
>
> —Heart recipient three years
> after transplant

"The way things work," Dr. Frist explains to the new transplant candidate, "we'll get you a beeper to wear so I can get in touch with you 24 hours a day." As soon as a heart's located, he says, "I would call you up and say, 'Come on to the hospital,' and that would be it."

Except that sometimes on final examination doctors find the donor's heart somehow defective or an inexact match with the recipient's tissue type. False alarms are another agony of waiting, along with the very fact of being tethered to that beeper because, once a heart is located, doctors may have as few as four hours before they must start the operation (see "Operation, The," below).

No one knows how long you'll have to wait, although many groups say the average is around 40 days. Obviously, the longer the wait the more exquisite the agony. Yet some recipients and families report unease at *not* having to wait at least long enough to get used to the idea.* "I checked in at noon on Friday," Mr. M said. "Saturday morning they said, 'You can't eat anything today because you may have surgery.' I'm saying, 'Hey! You guys told me it might be weeks. I'm not ready for this.'"

The reaction in a family can be mixed. Just three days after UCLA had approved Mr. O for its program, his wife says,

> We were sitting on the patio, and the phone rang. It was Suzanne, the coordinator. "Nick," she says, "I have a heart for you."
>
> We thought we'd have to wait at least three weeks, not three days. All I could think of was, "No, this is too soon. He's finally feeling well enough to move around a little. Let me have him for a few weeks before you stick him back in the hospital and take his heart away from him. I just don't want this now."
>
> But Nick's all excited, "Let's go! Let's get the bags packed!" And I'm thinking, "No! I don't want this." I was not going to tell him what I was feeling, but I was panicked. . . .

---

* Much turns on the patient's condition. Although Arthur Schoenberg had a very low priority because of his age, a heart that matched him, and no one else on the list, became available the day after UCLA admitted him to their program. We were all gratefully delighted because he hovered so near death that it did not appear he could wait even a week.

Still, most agree that the longer the wait, the harder it is. Almost inevitably, under such stress, you get on each other's nerves. Moreover, deterioration sets in. Mr. W suffered through four years of cardiomyopathy, with a seven-week wait once he was on the list at Vanderbilt. Mrs. W says:

> I'd sit across the table and look at him and see him going down, day to day; it's sad and hard. It got so bad at times, it was driving him crazy. He had no knowledge of what he was saying to me at times. And there were times I couldn't walk across the floor to please him. There was nothing I could do to help him; you just feel so helpless.
>
> Our marriage was hard to cope with, because of illness. Trying to understand each other, and couldn't, and knowing he was going down from day to day.

That likely deterioration, during a long wait, creates another role for the family: you must vigilantly monitor the patient's condition and intervene when necessary. Mrs. W continues:

> There were times he was so sick, and couldn't get his breath, I'd beg him to go to the doctor: "I'm not that sick. I'm not that bad." There were times I had to say very ugly things to him to get him to understand he was sick, and to get him to the hospital.

Similarly, you must guard against patients' tendency to buck up the people they love, to not "alarm" them. Dr. J. Kent Trinkle, head of cardiothoracic surgery at the University of Texas Health Science Center, San Antonio, says that all too often spouses "each will try to take me aside separately and say, 'Please don't mention the details: I don't want him (or her) to worry.'" That's when Dr. Trinkle sits them both down, together, and explains the situation fully; hidden truths can only become sources of worry, whereas people can handle even grim facts completely explained. "People will shut out the doctor's words when they have heard all they can handle," says Dr. Trinkle, "but they won't disintegrate emotionally."

But if a doctor doesn't intervene, you have to be alert to that protective tendency. "You had to learn to read between the lines," says one woman at a group meeting in Louisville. "John's face would turn blue, and I'd fight him: 'There's nothing wrong with me, I just can't breathe very well today.' I'd get him to the emergency room, and he'd still say, 'I'm doin' just fine! I'll be all right; just give me a little while.'"

"He's supporting her," says another wife.

"That's right," says Ruth Lusk, transplant coordinator at Humana.

"I think they all do that," adds the second wife.

You must be wary, and be there for them. Yet there's a catch. "There are times that you need to be by yourself," says the Humana group member who's waiting for a heart. "You need to go away, and close your door and just be entirely by yourself." Why? "I don't know, sometimes I feel like I want to go lay down, I want to cry. OK? In front of your family, you are putting up a front. Sometimes I can't any more; I've just got to be by myself, and get it out. If I cry in front of the kids—"

"They'll be crying in my office the next day!" says Ruth Lusk to a round of knowing laughter.

The woman waiting for the heart understands the problem that her occasional need for solitude can create. "That's kind of hard for your husband or wife or kids or anyone to see because, you know, if you go in there and close the door, their first reaction is to come in and see what's wrong with you."

"Yeah!" interjects her daughter. Understandably, because one sign of a need for intervention is unusual behavior patterns. The occasions can be overt, like the time, one Easter, when this woman assured everyone she was fine, then wished her son Happy Halloween (her medication needed adjustment). They can also be subtle. "You have to learn to pick up on signs, actions, just little things," says one family member. Like a usually hearty eater picking at dinner or an extrovert suddenly grown quiet. Or, sometimes, a retreat behind closed doors. The situation calls for fine-tuned judgment and sensitivity.

When her husband had so much trouble breathing, and was home alone all day because she worked, the Humana group wife told him, "If you feel like talking, you call us—we're not bothering you. I'll call periodically to say, 'Is everything OK?'; and you say, 'Uh-huh'—and hang up." She explained to the group, "I couldn't see putting him through having anybody stay with him because he had to feel like he was on his own."

"That's true," says the woman waiting for a heart, "you have to feel like you're doing for yourself." Her 15-year-old son reconciles the competing needs for monitoring and occasional privacy with particular neatness. "If I go in and lie down," she says, "he might come to the door and he's saying, 'Mom, I'm right in here if you need me.' Like, I'm here, but I know you want to be by yourself."

That's exactly the right spirit for the entire family.

For the rest, you must try to maintain as much activity as possible, especially any that specifically looks forward to a brighter future. Humana, for example, urges transplant candidates to start exercising, while still waiting, in what's usually a postoperative rehabilitation program. It helps fill the day, builds up their strength and circulation, and helps take them out of themselves, dwelling on illness. "Like with my husband," says one of the Humana group. "If he'd get depressed, I'd say, 'Hey! Just remember, we're gonna go on our cruise; you can't give up. Let's keep going!' We'd try to look forward to different things. We'd go out to eat once a month, everybody in the whole family—things like that."

Operation, The

Considering the drama of its circumstances and aftermath, a heart transplant is really a relatively simple operation. When doctors declare a potential donor brain dead, they maintain the body on life support machines as long as possible to supply all usable organs with oxygen until a recipient whose blood and tissue types match can be notified and prepared for transplant. When everything's set, surgeons remove the heart (and other organs) and flush it with an ice-cold solution to stop muscle activity and preserve the tissue. They pack it in ice and send it off in a Thermos unit (often by helicopter) to the hospital where the recipient waits. Speed is necessary because the heart, once cut from its blood supply, starts to deteriorate after four hours or so.*

Meanwhile, surgeons prepare the recipient as for a bypass operation. They open the chest and put the recipient on a heart-lung machine, stopping the diseased heart. They cut away all but the backs of the two atria, keeping the connections to the vena cava (which brings blood from the head and arms to the right atrium) and the pulmonary vein (which brings blood from the lungs to the left atrium). They cut the recipient's aorta and pulmonary artery just above their respective valves. They remove the old heart, often sending it to the lab to help researchers further determine the causes and mechanics of heart disease.

Now surgeons stitch the new heart (minus, of course, the two atrial backs) onto what is left of the old heart, also connecting up the aorta and pulmonary artery. With a catheter in the left atrium, they flush the left heart with a saline solution to remove all air before they finally sew the last stitches.

When they remove clamps from the veins and arteries, and take the recipient off the heart-lung machine, the new heart almost always

---

* Right now, researchers in California are testing a device, about the size of a TV set, that they think can keep the heart beating and fresh for up to 72 hours after removal from the donor's body. So far it's worked with the hearts of sheep, pigs, and dogs for 24 hours.

starts beating on its own. If not, the surgeons start it with a mild shock. They close, and the recipient starts life over.

However "simple," a transplant does require a lot of steps, and generally takes five or so hours. During that time the family will get (or should seek out, see chapter 6) progress reports, same as with a bypass.

Operation, After the

Most of the recovery is as for bypass or any other major surgery (see chapter 7). But a few new wrinkles appear.

Start with the plus side. Like any patients hit by the 10-ton truck called major surgery, transplant recipients look awful for hours afterward. But—if whatever condition led them to transplant involved drastically bad circulation, they may look *better* (if you ignore the tubes coming out of them) than they did immediately before. No more distressing gray look.

The down side of this phenomenon is psychological. "I was weaker than hell," one recipient said. "I thought, I have a new heart, so why can't I just get up and, like, run?" Because all of the debilitations that plagued the patient before the transplant still rule the body. Yes, the muscles now get enough blood; but that perfusion alone does not cure the atrophy they suffered while weakness kept their owner prostrate. They need rebuilding.

The point is—one the family should pound home—now those muscles *can* be built up; their residual weakness, despite the new heart, constitutes a challenge, not cause for depression.

The only other phenomenon peculiar to transplants are two of the side effects of anti-rejection medication: puffiness, especially in the face, which is common; and hair growth in inappropriate places, somewhat rarer. Both are disconcerting for anyone; for those keenly concerned with their looks, they can be devastating. The family might offer two calming thoughts. First, as with the disadvantages of old age, consider the alternative. Better still, the side effects diminish with the size of the doses, then generally disappear. Surely a trifling price to pay.

Questions, Most Often Asked

Strangely enough, according to Dr. Roland Girardet, these do not include "How long will I live?" Why not? "Because," Dr. Girardet says, "they don't expect to live long. They probably dare not ask; they're afraid of the answer. So I tell them the statistics." These vary from center to center, but 77% of all recipients since the introduction of cyclosporine were going strong *five years* after their transplants.

What questions do patients mostly ask Dr. Girardet? "How will I be able to function after the transplant? Will I be an invalid? or will I be able to work? function like a human being?" His answer: "You'll be able to do anything you want, anything you did before and would like to do—if things go well." As we see throughout this book, how well things go depends to a surprising degree on the patient, therefore on the family's encouragement and cooperation.

Another usual set of questions, Dr. Girardet says, relates to quality of life. His answer is the same: assuming normal recovery, they can do literally what they like. "I'm not sure they believe me," adds Dr. Girardet with a smile. "But it's true."

Other common questions (page references in parentheses if they're also answered in detail elsewhere in the book):

Q: Can I hope to feel good, ever, considering how bad I feel now, pre-operation?

A: Absolutely (p. 52, "Condition," above).

Q: (Immediately post-op) The regimen is so crowded, will I ever do anything except watch medication, have biopsies, and so on?

A: Of course. The regimen slackens with recovery.

Q: (Especially from spouses, when told that at first they must monitor the taking of medications) There are so many, can I keep track of them?

A: (From patient's wife) "I ask people who ask me that, 'What are *you* taking now?' And they're on this and this—four or five pills, themselves. 'Well,' I say, 'do you mind that?' No, it's routine. So I say, 'Well?'"

They think it's going to be the biggest chore they've ever had in their lives, to get these medicines into the patient. But when they realize they've taken theirs on time for 10 years, they can handle it."

Make a chart of medications, photocopy it, and check off each dose, each time it's taken. (See sample chart on page 111.)

Q: (The wife of a longtime recipient relays what she hears from "newcomers") "They ask, 'Will he be in a wheelchair? For how long? How long before he can go outside?' I'm sure the doctors and nurses have told them. But they always want to know, 'When did Jack go out?'"

A: The exact timing is irrelevant (see p. 93, "Length of Stay," chapter 7). The point is, Jack *did* and so, in all likelihood, will the one you're worried about.

Q: (Immediately post-op) With all the warnings about the danger of infection, and family having to wear gowns and masks to visit, do patients have to live in some sterile environment for an extended period?

A: No. Once they go home, they avoid people with colds, avoid crowds, and wear a surgical mask when they go out in a crowd, but only for the first few months.

Q: How long in the hospital?

A: (1) Dr. Frist: "Anywhere from 10 days minimum, to six weeks. Everyone has *some* rejection and infection; it depends on how bad." (2) p. 93 (chapter 7 again).

Q: Still feel bad after the operation?

A: Yes and No. Yes, remember that 10-ton truck and months, maybe years, of debilitation and atrophy (p. 60, "Operation, After the," above). No, whatever problems you had solely because of no blood supply—angina, trouble breathing, difficulty eating, etc.—poof! are gone! And the "yes" part yields to time and effort.

Q: (Pre-op) With all this talk of AIDS, should patients (1) donate their own blood? (2) enlist donors they trust?

A: (1) Depending on your condition, they probably wouldn't take it; if they would, it has to be frozen because fresh blood lasts only 42 days. (2) Sure, if it makes you feel better; besides, hospitals need all the donations they can get. But, in fact, screening today is rigorous.

Questions, "Stupid"

The only stupid question is one that you don't ask, the one you hide within yourself and worry about.

—Dr. William DeVries

Yes, yes. But who's going to "bother" a busy doctor or nurse with questions about, say, washing hands? You'd sound stupid. So, instead, you just fret about it. Mrs. J, whose husband received a transplant three years ago, runs into that all the time counseling the families of new recipients:

One wife was worried about how she was going to get her husband's hands washed if they went out to eat; those bathrooms aren't very sanitary. I said, 'Well, carry a Wipette in your purse for him.' She hadn't asked anyone before because she thought that was a stupid question, but her mind was relieved. She hadn't thought about that. She probably would have by the time they'd gone out a few times.

Maybe. Then, again, maybe she would have worried enough so that they didn't go out and missed that stimulus of a return to normal living.

The same woman regularly fields "stupid" questions about taking the vital anti-rejection drug, cyclosporine. Wives say to her, "Well, we can't go anywhere; we have to be *home* at nine o'clock to take rejection medicine." She tells them, "Nonsense; just tote along a small can or bottle of juice." She once went out to dinner with five recent transplant couples and insisted they follow her lead, measuring and mixing the cyclosporine and juice at the table. "Two ladies have since said, 'I never would have put it on the table. I would have thought it was offensive to other people.' And I said, 'So what? It's your life-line!'" (Although she's plainly right, you can avoid the issue by taking along a pre-measured dose in a small bottle, which you unobtrusively add to mild or juice.)

The 15-year-old son of a woman about to receive a transplant of heart and lungs finally mustered courage enough to ask his father, "Will Mom still love me, with a new heart?" Can you imagine the possible problems if, instead of asking, he had simply brooded? But he was still a youngster, you say, and maybe unsophisticated? What adult would think such things? A lawyer in his late 30s, after his transplant, ended a marriage that had floundered for years. Reacting to many long-building stresses, he says he went "hog wild," with drunken binges and a 19-year-old girlfriend. And what did his friends and legal associates think? "He's got a 17-year-old heart."

The only stupid question, the only ones that can cause trouble, are the ones you don't ask. Make sure your whole family, the patient included, understands that essential fact.

Recovery, Long-term

The recovery of the transplant recipient we know best, Arthur Schoenberg, has been so marvelous we may have a distortedly rosy view of this: not of the realistic possibilities, but of the reality many seem to face.

This thought struck when, in Ottawa, a social worker complained that so many transplant recipients "are sitting and watching the rain fall; they're depressed." He says that the majority have not returned to work; many of the men remain impotent. A nurse in San Antonio says, "I'm not certain that all of the time with all of the patients the quality of life *is* that good after their transplant." Their physical problems—the angina, shortness of breath, weakness—they disappear but the recipients often trade one set of illnesses for another, including high blood pressure, diabetes, muscle cramps, and psychological problems. She wonders if, perhaps, they should put more stress on "the realities of the transplant."

Our first reaction, shaped by our unqualified joy over Arthur, was, *What* "realities"? Everything's wonderful!

Of course we know not every case is a triumph. One poor soul tells us, "My life is on hold. I'm waiting for him to die. I just wonder how much longer he can handle the pain and deterioration." But that was medical: her husband had an undiagnosed, incurable condition of the spleen that, detected, would have ruled out the transplant. At UCLA, which has an outstanding survival record, four of the first 110 patients died of acute rejection; but significantly, two of those simply would not comply with doctors' orders, a matter of attitude. But unless some unexpected condition complicates matters, transplant patients face only one specific disability connected to the operation: because doctors must sever some nerves, the heart rate lags when they exercise and does not return to normal as quickly. Big deal! So they have to warm up and cool off more. A matter of attitude. Indeed, we're convinced that absent some specific medical dishevelment, a transplant recipient's course of recovery and quality of life turn on his or her attitude.

That may depend on what preceded the transplant. We've bragged about the smoothness of Arthur Schoenberg's recovery. But in fact, he suffered a small stroke during the operation, leaving a slight droop to one eyelid and some impairment of his left hand's strength; he had the usual episodes of rejection and infection, the characteristic puffiness of those anti-rejection drugs—no worse, but no less. Why does he surmount all that and relish his life when others "watch the rain fall?" Of course, part is surely character; he had always been a fighter and a perfect patient. But another factor also counts. After 20 years of living with a heart condition, Arthur had deteriorated so far that he anticipated the end with resigned dignity. The very possibility of transplant came as an astonishment, the fact that it happened, a near miracle.* For Arthur, every moment since has been golden, a bonus.

We understand how different it might be for younger people or for those who had not suffered particular ravages of heart disease too much before. Those who make fine recoveries see the medicine, the biopsies, any restrictions of diet or activity as a trifle compared with how they felt and what they faced before. That regimen may grind the spirits of others who cannot stop pining for the carefree health they enjoyed before the onset of disease. For them, cyclosporine is a burden, not a blessing. For them, the necessary disciplines of perpetual post-transplant therapy make life a prison, not a boon.

---

* We cannot let slip this opportunity to publicly thank Dr. Phil Marcus, long a dear friend, who insisted that Arthur's age might not be the absolute barrier we supposed. Without Phil, it would not have happened.

What can you and the family do to help? It starts with a negative, what *not* to do. As Dr. Kent Trinkle observes, "when serious illness strikes, some families will withdraw from the patient; they seem to want to distance themselves before the inevitable pain sets in." Alternatively, they smother the patient with attention. Dr. Trinkle urges families to treat their patient as naturally and honestly as they did before a problem developed. "No *special* treatment," Dr. Trinkle insists, "is the kindest treatment of all."

For what you can do, positively, harken to Bobbie Scallorn, at San Antonio's Audie L. Murphy VA Hospital, the nurse who spoke of transplant's realities:

> Some transplant patients have given up control of their lives: their jobs, handling the check book, giving advice to family members, decision-making. And now they've got somebody telling them when to have an appointment, when to take their medicine. The more they've given up, the more depressed and the more they don't care. The family starts feeding on this and it becomes a real dynamic problem.
>
> That's what I'm seeing—like in one of my transplant patients. I feel if he could take over his business again, some of the authority, he would do better. He denies that's why he's depressed; he'll tell you that he and his wife decided before the transplant that this is the way it's going to be. Well, this is *after* the transplant and he needs to *get on with his life*! He needs to take back control.
>
> It's really important for the family to encourage the person to *be* well: "You've had your transplant, now it's time to *live*. If something happens, we'll deal with it when it happens. Don't wait for it to happen."
>
> Until we get the families turned around to help the patients get back, I don't think it's going to change.

When patients get the right support, and have the right attitude, the result is wonderful. When someone commented that many people automatically figure transplant patients are incapacitated, a nurse said about two of her prize transplants, "That's exactly why people like Al and Jimmy are so adamant about doing things like triathalons—to show people. They want to let people know they aren't sitting around. Some transplants get into playing the sick role, and they can't get out of it. It's just a habit: they sit around and think they really *are* sick. Jimmy wanted to skydive; but they wouldn't let him. So he rappels down buildings, he climbs rocks, he does rescue work."*

---

* A final brag about Arthur. As soon as he was back on his feet, he insisted on turning in his state handicapped parking placard. "I am not," he said firmly, "handicapped."

The family's message in word, deed, and attitude must be a slight amendment to the way Bobbie Scallorn put it: "This is *after* the transplant and you need to *get on with your life*—because we need and want you the way you were and now can be again"!

CHAPTER 6

Facing Surgery*

Attitude Going In

The best prescription we've heard comes from Dr. Alan Lansing, director of Humana Heart Institute, International in Louisville:

> People should not undergo an operative procedure they don't believe in. They may be frightened; but they have to believe that this is right for them or that the procedure is necessary, that they *must* have it. They should not be forced into something that they think is wrong for them.

That means faith in the medical people involved, and faith in the institution where the operation will take place. It means feeling comfortable about asking questions, feeling sure of getting answers.

Of course you may ask questions against a backdrop of generally excellent care that (again generally) keeps improving. As you saw on page 6, Dr. William DeVries marvels at advances in coronary surgery even since 1975, with operations that then threatened a one-in-four mortality rate now being 99% successful.

Better techniques in anesthesia, monitoring, ways of lowering body temperature so that the heart and other organs require less oxygen, support devices like the intraaortic pump to help postoperative

---

* Or angioplasty or anything they call "a procedure." As we wrote before, whenever anyone wants to put anything in you except food or drink, and especially if they propose to make a new opening to do it, ask questions.

circulation—all manner of advances contribute to greater safety and greater assurance.

Still you should ask questions, starting with this basic one:

IS THIS PROCEDURE NECESSARY?

Then you follow up: What are the alternatives? For instance, is angioplasty possible instead of bypass? Medication instead of angioplasty? What if we do nothing? In all cases, what risks balance the benefits?

Other follow-up questions may strike you as impertinent or downright impolite. They are necessary exactly because medicine advances so fast and so far nowadays. You must ask whether the answers you got to the first set of questions represent the latest or majority medical opinion. For instance, doctors routinely order angioplasties after treatment with the clot-dissolver, TPA. But an extensive 1988 study demonstrated that a better course was to administer the clot-dissolver and simply wait to see if *this* case warranted angioplasty.

By the time patient and family go through the litany of these questions and answers, all can go ahead with confidence in whatever the decision. That is the only right attitude for facing any procedure.

Doctor, Choosing a (Also see all other "Doctor" listings, and "Hospital, Choosing a," below)

This is an advanced exercise in "Yes, but . . ." You want the best medical help available for someone you love. Therefore you always choose the most competent, most experienced doctor available, don't you? Yes, but . . . suppose the patient (or you) simply cannot communicate with that doctor. Yes, but . . . how about such issues as those discussed, below, in "Doctors, Matching, with Complexity of Case."

All right, then, you want someone with whom the entire family feels comfortable. Yes, but suppose this case presents complexities, and the best pair of hands in town belong to someone whose personality reminds you that it's time to defrost the refrigerator?

It gets complicated.

If you're likely to spend a lot of time with a doctor, especially if you must rely on that doctor for information about, and referrals to, other doctors—specialists, generally—the chemistry between the doctor and the patient, you, and the rest of the family is important. For a one-shot procedure, especially a complicated case, competence and experience outweigh charm and compatibility.

Everything being equal, look for the doctor who evidences interest in all of you as people. The husband of a woman who needed a transplant explained why they decided on Dr. William Frist at

Vanderbilt, after a lengthy search: "Out of all the specialists who had run tests, Dr. Frist was the first who ever called us. He was the only one we ever spoke to personally. And my wife made the statement, 'If someone's going to cut on me, I want to know him. I want to feel like they've got my best interest at heart.'"

Doctors, Matching, with Complexity of Case

When Mr. K had his heart attack eight years ago, his general practitioner was in the hospital recovering from an operation. Mrs. K drove Mr. K to the emergency room of a small community hospital. "It turned out," says Mrs. K, "that the doctor who's now Bob's cardiologist is the one they called. Very competent. Very good for the kind of treatment he needed, which wasn't dramatic."

Very sensible. They felt comfortable with him; it was a routine case that he treated with competent, concerned, personal interest for eight years. Then Mr. K's condition deteriorated enough to require a bypass. At that point their doctor, knowing his own limitations, referred them to a specialist.

Since the key is knowing how complex the case is, that should be one of your first questions. Is this a serious, difficult case or is it run-of-the-mill? Or somewhere in between? If it's complex, does the doctor's level of experience match the complexity? If you feel uncomfortable putting it in quite those challenging terms, simply ask if this doesn't require a specialist.

Plainly, for a difficult case, the central issue is finding someone who can handle it. But if the routinely high level of competence common today matches the routine nature of most cases, other considerations should prevail. Dr. Sam Teichman explains:

> It's only in the minority of very, very difficult cases where you need the physician who's recommended as God's gift to humanity because he or she is so brilliant.
>
> You need somebody who knows what he's doing, but there are many gradations between doctors who see 20 heart attacks a year, those who see 200, and those who see 2000. If you've got a routine case, 200 is enough for them to be experienced and comfortable. Then what's important is if they're going to take the time to explain everything and make *you* feel comfortable.
>
> You don't need the experts who see 2000 cases if they don't have the time to talk to the patient, to the family, to explain what's going on and offer comfort.

Although it sounds almost sacrilegious to say that you don't need or want "the best" for someone you love, that may often be the case.

As Dr. Teichman puts it, "Families feel, 'Oh my God! Dad is having a heart attack; we have to get him the absolute best cardiologist, most expensive, most exclusive, most difficult to reach.'" In other words, someone s who's essentially too busy to take the case, and who, if it is routine, may consider it almost beneath notice. "I think that's inappropriate," says Dr. Teichman.

You should think so, too.

Doctors, Referrals from and to

Few patients get to a surgeon or any other specialist on their own;* almost all are referred: from a general practitioner to a cardiologist; from a cardiologist to a surgeon; and so on. You want to be sure that the person you love is in good hands. Should you simply take the referral, salute, and trot off to make an appointment?

"It goes without saying," says Dr. Simon Stertzer, "that your confidence in the first level of advice is critical." A physician obviously can locate and evaluate talent and experience in another physician far better than lay people. Of course, you have to trust *your* doctor, assume that he or she has no ax to grind, and is interested exclusively in the patient's welfare.

Ideally, that mindset should animate all referrals. "Realistically," says Dr. Stertzer, "the average GP or internist will say, 'I use so-and-so as my cardiologist; I like him, I know him, he doesn't steal my patients, he and I are at the same golf club.'" That isn't necessarily bad. "Fortunately," Dr. Stertzer continues, "the training of medical personnel in the United States is generally good enough so in most cases it won't matter; we have a pretty high standard of care with referrals made on a personal basis." The principle of "Doctors, Matching, etc.," above, applies.

Even so, and even if this appears to be one of the routine cases, your family's best interests are served by asking more questions. It is your right, even your duty. "People are intimidated by physicians," says Dr. Sam Teichman. "They shouldn't allow themselves to be. An internist says, 'Don't worry, I've called a cardiologist who'll take care of it.' They should stop and say, tactfully and respectfully, 'Why'd you pick that one? Explain. Is he the best? In what way? Is there anyone else we should consider? For what reasons?'"

Dr. Stertzer suggests some appropriate answers: "Your doctor tells you, 'Well, this guy started this procedure.' Or, 'He has done 5,000.'

---

* But see the exception in "Negotiating Fees," below.

Or, 'He is a recognized expert.' Or, 'If *I* needed this procedure, I would go to *him.*'"

Just remember that an equally valid response is, "This is someone I've known and used with great success for years, someone with more than enough experience for your quite routine case, and someone who cares, whom I think you'll find *sympatico,* and who will take the time to explain everything to you."

Doctors, Second Opinions from

Dr. John Hutchinson, a renowned surgeon in New Jersey, finds that most patients are remarkably knowledgeable about their condition by the time he sees them because they've already talked to a number of doctors about it: "They've been through diagnosis several times," he says, "because insurance companies require second opinions."

The insurance industry's interest, in this case, is the same as yours: they want to be sure an operation is necessary before they pay for any of it. It may not be. In 1988, the RAND Corporation, a California think tank, studied 386 bypass cases at three hospitals. RAND called 14% of the surgeries "inappropriate," and found another 30% "equivocal"; they considered only 56% plainly justified. The study's physician-authors said that "It . . . emphasizes the need for patients to question their doctors closely and seek second opinions . . ."

Understand, a doctor who suggests an operation other doctors pronounce unnecessary is not necessarily wrong. In the science of medicine, diagnosis and prescription remain, largely, arts. So proper treatment often remains a matter of opinion, the precise reason insurance companies generally mandate second (or more) opinions before they shell out, and why you should generally insist on getting them.

You and the insurance industry part company when the first doctor denies a need for more radical treatment—*if* the lesser treatment doesn't seem to do the job.

The wife of Dr. Manuel Straker, a Los Angeles psychiatrist, had suffered for years from a defective heart valve, the result of childhood rheumatic fever. The Strakers brought up the possibility of surgery with their cardiologist, who explained why he found it inappropriate: the valve was certainly repairable, but he thought the heart muscle by now so damaged as to bar her as a candidate for surgery.

Arrhythmias grew worse and culminated in an incident of cardiac arrest. Now desperate, the Strakers again asked about surgery. As Dr. Straker explains:

Our treating doctor still thought he might be able to control the arrhythmia by the use of medication and so on. *However, we did insist on getting another opinion.* The new cardiologist had additional information and additional training, particularly in control of arrhythmias. He encouraged us, in fact insisted, that we get her to a cardiac surgeon as soon as possible. Otherwise she was very unlikely to survive even three or four months.

When they operated, they found that the heart muscle was, in fact, much stronger than anyone had hoped. They repaired the valve and Mrs. Straker has made, Dr. Straker says, "a wonderful kind of recovery." He goes on:

If there's something to be learned from this it's that no matter how skillful the doctor is, it's always useful to have a second opinion or a third opinion. That's very important.

And it's also extremely important not to give up hope, not to accept what seems to be inevitable as though it were in fact inevitable. Make every effort to deal with the problem in any way that's more constructive than simply accepting it and giving up.

All that is so patently sensible no one can argue. But, in practice, doubts often assail patients and, even more, families. Won't the doctor be annoyed if we ask for another opinion? You know that old joke:

Doctor: You're grossly overweight.
Patient: I want a second opinion.
Doctor: OK, you're ugly.

Isn't asking for a second opinion as much as saying, "We don't trust you?" If we ask, mightn't the doctor "take it out" on the patient? Or just lose interest and no longer try as hard? Quite the contrary. As Dr. Sam Teichman puts it:

Family members have to assume the doctors' honor and motives are right. I've seen the attitude that, "Maybe if I offend them they'll spend less time or not care as much." But I'd say it's totally unjustifiable.

He assures us that no competent and confident doctor will mind your request for a second opinion. Peer reviews are routine in the profession precisely because so much is a matter of opinion. Indeed, Dr. Teichman says, if a physician is so insecure about a second opinion, "it would worry *me.*"

Who should pick the reviewing doctor or doctors? It doesn't much matter: the original doctor, the chief of that department at the hospital, someone your research has revealed as expert; many hospitals have "patient advocates" or ombudsmen who can make suggestions. But, of course, you may want a second opinion even about that.

Doctors, Switching

Start with the easy part: the reasons you should *not* switch doctors. Leading the list is the possibility that you or the rest of the family don't like the doctor as a matter of personality or chemistry, not competence. So what? If the patient is plainly "in good hands," it does not really matter that you might not want to shake one of them. That was the case with Mrs. N, who says:

> I had a really bad relationship with my husband's doctor. He had been my doctor, too, and I had left him because I didn't like him. But Pete had stayed with him. They went to college together; they were "old buddies."
>
> Well, he really had Pete's best interest in mind and he brought in all the best specialists and everything. I guess he's fine as a doctor; it's his personality I can't stand. I just don't *relate* well to him. But my husband likes him and has confidence in him, and that's what counts.

Actually, "liking" shouldn't have counted much even with the patient; "confidence" is the key, especially if the doctor is one of the specialists with whom you hope to have few, if decisively helpful, dealings. Reverse the situation and the point makes itself: your whole family may count some doctor among your warmest friends, but if he or she plainly isn't doing the job, you want someone else.

The next reason for *not* switching doctors is an attempt to "trade up" to better results. Alice has been pleased with the way their cardiologist has controlled her husband's angina—until Zachary mentions that his wife's doctor has her on nitroglycerin patches instead of pills, a treatment that seems to have virtually ended the problem. The exchange leaves Zachary feeling pretty smug until Bart hails the genius of his father's doctor for having *literally* ended angina with a bypass. Then Yolanda deflates Bart with an account of how her brother's doctor achieved the same results without an operation, using angioplasty instead.

If you want the results enjoyed by someone else's spouse, parent, sibling, friend, etc., you need that etc. whose heart condition exhibits those particular complexities and severities, not those patients' doctors. There are not only no miracles involved in the treatment of any heart condition (at least none you can count on or obtain through a cunning choice of doctors); there are also no particular mysteries or secrets.

It is fashionable to say "Medicine is an art," which is largely true; what is untrue is to finish the catch phrase with "not a science." Medicine is both art and science. That means it has definite rules, definitive tests, standard procedures. Different doctors prescribe different treatments for different heart patients because—surprise—

the patients are different. Even when their conditions bear the same label—"angina," "coronary occlusion," "valve stenosis," etc.—they can differ so widely in severity, complication, prognosis, and in the patient's overall condition, that the wonder is not that treatments (and their results) differ, but that they are at all similar (also see "Fads," below).

All this, of course, is in the context of questioning, confidence, and second opinions as discussed above. Given all that, though, switching doctors because some other doctor's patient seems to be doing better is folly.

Then when should you switch?

We've already covered lack of confidence in the doctor's ability or unwillingness to solicit additional opinion, especially if recovery, progress, or prognosis is poor. Add to those reasons even the *slightest* tendency in a doctor to a cavalier attitude toward the patient's condition. If some night your patient has chest pain and you call the doctor only to hear some variation on the theme of "Take two aspirin and call me in the morning" (most common is, "Oh, it's probably gas or maybe a slight kidney reaction; we'll check it out at my office— *tomorrow*) start looking for another doctor, and don't wait for morning. Even if it turns out that, yes, this time it was just a little gas or whatever, you still need a doctor who does not diagnose by mental telepathy or practice long-distance medicine, who would rather answer false alarms than ever be late for a single fire. Of course, you have a responsibility to consciously avoid crying wolf. But anyone dealing with heart conditions who objects to being yanked out of bed should consider switching specialties.

We saved the most common impetus to switching doctors for last. Dr. William DeVries says that the central question to ask yourself when selecting a doctor, especially for primary care, is: "Can I communicate? Is this doctor going to listen to me? talk to me? answer my questions? If not, you need to go to someone who will."

Communication occupies the position of first importance in the relationship. Ask Dr. Sam Teichman what the family can do to best help their patient recover, and he tells you:

> They should ask questions to the point where they understand what's going on. If a physician is unwilling or unable to explain what it is he or she is thinking or doing, it's time to find another physician.

Fads

When someone you love is ill, you're naturally alive to the least hint of any "cure." Especially if the regimen doctors propose is long and hard, it's human to snatch at any suggestion of something that's easy, a "magic bullet" or "miracle cure." That's the secret of the diet books that chase each other relentlessly on and off of the bestseller list. Who wants to cut calories rigorously and continuously and eat sensibly when "all you have to do is . . ." whatever this week's sensation prescribes?

Mrs. B's husband underwent a quadruple bypass, ending three years of angina pain. He made a marvelous recovery. But Mrs. B remains mightily annoyed. She read a book, afterward. Now she says, "Dr._____ does *not* recommend the surgery; let's say he does not advocate bypass surgery; he feels you should do it with exercise and diet. You should change your diet to unblock; he strongly feels that people can do it through diet, and that only with a much smaller percentage is heart surgery really required."

Well, isn't that the point we made about the RAND study in "Doctors, Second Opinions from," above? Not at all. The point there was that you should have more than one opinion. Mr. and Mrs. B got *three* opinions, unanimous for bypass, but because of that book Mrs. B still says, "You wonder, 'Were you rushed into it?'" Thank goodness she read the book *after* the surgery.

"We run into this all the time," says Dr. Allan Lansing, "when we talk to patients and families." He continues:

> They've heard about vitamin E or fish oil or whatever the latest fad may be. And I recognize that for the occasional person some of these things may be beneficial; but you have to try to give the patient and family perspective on where *this* patient stands.
>
> If somebody has a left main coronary lesion,* and is saying, "If I just exercise and have the right diet and so on I'll be all right," then you have to talk about how threatening this is.
>
> If people still don't listen, if they're still convinced by what they read in some magazine or what Aunt Suzy said, you've done all you can.

Quackery is not necessarily at issue; diet and exercise may be just the ticket for some patients—as, indeed, they form part of the regimen for nearly all. But prescriptions and proscriptions should come *only* from examining doctors. Your doctor may not always "know best," but he or she assuredly knows better for *this* patient than does the author of Mrs. B's book or Aunt Suzy *or* Aunt Suzy's doctor.

Does that make the author of Mrs. B's book (or Aunt Suzy) a villain? No. "People have to ride a hobby horse," Dr. Lansing says,

---

* In fairness, Mrs. B's book did allow that left main blockage absolutely requires surgery.

generously, "because that's the only way you get anybody's attention; but the hobby horse isn't good for everybody."

There's nothing wrong with asking any attending doctor about any treatment you've read or heard about, so long as you attend to the answer about its wisdom for *this* patient, and remember that rejection does not signal the doctor's part in a medical-fraternity conspiracy to suppress a cure so simple it would drive them all out of business. The instances fanatics adduce of treatments, once thought eccentric or sham, that are now standard do not somehow "prove" the worth of *this* one. Science demands long, documented, clinical proof. And for every Lister and Pasteur, hundreds purvey monkey glands and peach pits.

Family, Role of the

Doctor Leon Resnekov calls preparation for surgery "an insoluble problem without love and support in the family." He says, "I see it over and over, all sorts of doubts and fears in the patient's mind. I think physicians sometimes make a big mistake by not talking about these things before surgery."

Your role is to make sure that all doubts and fears are fully ventilated. It may mean forcing the issue. If your patient is reticent or uneasy about expressing emotions, you must surface the questions. If medical people are not easily forthcoming, you must play the ombudsman, commanding dialogue. You must enlist the family's participation, rally their support.

With most of the family, participation is more vital than decision. Mrs. W, in Tennessee, had to decide whether to risk a heart/lung transplant immediately or try to survive as best, and long, as she could without it. She decided to go ahead, and says:

> The family was real supportive. They reassured me. It helped a whole lot to know that your family was backing you. The decision was up to me and my husband, but they told me how they felt about it. You couldn't make a decision like that all on your own without consulting your family.

The family's support afterward will be all the greater because they were consulted before.

One vital area of decision before any major surgery, especially for a heart condition, is a mature facing of the fact that something can go wrong. If it does, no one will be in emotional shape to make certain decisions; patients generally cannot then make their wishes known. The time to talk over the patient's desires is beforehand.

How do they feel about long-term life-support systems? What kind of heroic measures do they want taken? What are the emotional and financial implications?

Infection sent Mr. H into a coma after a *second* heart transplant. Mrs. H says that during those months, besides faith in their doctor,

> . . . what made it easier was Jim and I had talked, so I knew what he wanted. That made any decision that I had to make easier. And I'd advise any family: always talk and be prepared ahead of time. If it came to the point, I could have made the decision easier because I *knew* what Jim wanted rather than just guessing at it.

Mrs. H demonstrated another prime family role. It was she who noticed the signs of disorientation that heralded her husband's coma; she got him to the hospital just in time. If someone is awaiting surgery, again especially with a heart condition, chances are the condition is serious enough so that instant action is essential whenever they appear to "go sour." It's up to the family, those who know the patient best, to spot the signs—generally any abnormal behavior, like sudden lethargy, quiet, depression, lack of appetite, sleeplessness—and *do* something.

Beyond that, as Dr. Allan Lansing says when asked what the family can do to help the surgeon, "I would like them to take as much of a positive attitude as possible about the future." For the present, Dr. Lansing says:

> What the family can do, basically, is relieve concern that the patient might have about the welfare of other members of the family—things like, "How will everyone manage"; or "What's going to happen to the farm while I'm away." And so on.
>
> They need to talk about good things, positive things that are going on in the family, and how they're taking care of any problems or worries the patient might have.

You can all, even distant family members, simply *be there* for the patient—if not always physically, by phone: it's important to *say*, "Now, be sure to call if you need me," and say it with conviction.

Finances and Insurance

In 1974, we wrote:

> Medical costs are not outrageous. They used to be outrageous 10 or 15 years ago; now they are simply impossible. Literally. Unless you are very rich or very poor, you flat-out cannot afford any major illness today. If you are poor enough to qualify, you can get excellent,

if often somewhat impersonal, medical attention, free.* If you're rich
enough, well . . . after the illness is over, you will be notably less
rich.

That was before the cost of health care went *up,* before the march of
technology made so many new (and expensive) procedures available—
like the $100,000 heart transplant, or the artificial devices that can cost
upwards of $200,000 a year, or even "ordinary" bypasses at $35,000
or so.

Between the extremes of rich and poor, most people rely on
insurance: Medicare, or their employer's group plan, or such private
insurance as Blue Cross and Blue Shield. What are the provisions of
a reasonable insurance policy? "A premium that's not ridiculous,"
says Jody Polk, account manager for the Cardiothoracic Group at
UCLA Medical Center, "and a deductible that's not ridiculous." A
standard policy covers 80% up to a certain amount, usually $5000–
$8000, then 100% of charges above that amount. It should have
minimal exclusions (i.e., conditions not covered), which should *not*
include heart conditions or cancer.

Even with reasonable policies, coverage terms can vary widely.
You should know ahead of time what your policy offers: how much
it allows for which services, particularly for elective surgery.

If someone you love needs something not covered—well, you will
manage. Even then, hospitals may cooperate, breaking up their
charges in ways that take advantage of what your insurance does
allow. Make such arrangements ahead of time. It is too late once a
charge has been submitted and turned down; even a tolerant insurance
company gives you only one try. Hospitals and doctors' offices tend
to be expert about insurance, protecting your rights to maximum
coverage (which after all may mean their right to be paid!); most have
someone who can answer your questions. Jody Polk advises starting
with the social services department, which virtually all hospitals have.
Have a copy of the policy in hand; even experts cannot explain terms
of a policy that is not there.

You must be sure the insurance remains in force, which means
thoroughly understanding its terms. If the policy derives from the
patient's employment, what happens during extended recovery?
Suppose the patient cannot return to work? On the other hand, if it's
your policy, what keeps it in force? Many wives, for instance, discover
they must keep working to protect their husband's coverage.

Then there's the question of family finances.

---

* See "Free Care," below.

Even if you normally handle the routine paying of bills and such, you now must be clear about *exactly* where your family stands financially so you can anticipate any changes that surgery may impel. If the patient is a wage earner, will that income continue? How long? If not, do you have enough other sources of income? Should you do anything now to assure the alternate income? Must you file insurance claims or state disability or workmen's compensation forms? Again, the hospital's social services people can probably advise.

In line with relieving the patient of worry, as we discussed above in "Family, Role of the," Dr. Shahbudin Rahimtoola says:

> I think you ought to start putting your house in order. If the husband has been handling all the finances, and he's the patient, the wife's got to educate herself, to be in a better position to cope and be self-sustaining. Not that she necessarily will have to go out and earn, but she's got to understand the total family finances. She has to be prepared to take over running many things.
>
> Certainly, there should be a will.

This is not morbidity. Even with routine procedures, attended by minimal risk, you should address such matters if only to relieve your patient's mind. The more serious the operation, the more urgent the need. "All of that being done," Dr. Rahimtoola says, "takes a load off the husband. He knows that she's going to be able to understand and cope. Otherwise, he's worried—he might not tell her, but he's *worried* about it."*

In all likelihood, so is she. "We went to see our accountant," says Mrs. N about the period before her husband's transplant. "I wanted to make sure our will was proper, the house was OK, and the deeds and everything were in order. I wanted to know that, if something happened, I wouldn't have to go through a state of panic."

Free Care (Also see "Finances and Insurance," above)

Almost no one can "afford" health care today. But if you have no insurance, are not eligible for Medicare or similar state programs, and have no money, you can still find excellent help.

Patients who served in the armed forces may qualify for a Veteran's Administration hospital. Check with any VA office for eligibility rules.

---

* The reverse situation is a husband assuring his patient-wife that he can run the house and care for the children (or has arranged for those functions) if he's never before shared them.

Federal legislation, the Hill-Burton Act, lets hospitals that have borrowed from the government pay back in services to the needy. Your state department of health can identify participating local hospitals.

Finally, you usually can find a nearby county hospital with no (or token) charges for those who cannot pay.

Do you get what you pay for? That is, not much—or nothing? No; you get much more. Jody Polk, accounting manager for the Cardiothoracic Group at UCLA, a private hospital, says this about county treatment: "The facilities aren't as nice; but as far as the care and competence of those physicians, it's absolutely equal. Doctors are doctors; you're going to find good and bad wherever you go."

Dr. Shahbudin Rahimtoola, whom we quote in these pages, is chief of cardiology at USC/County Medical Center in Los Angeles. You have only to examine his credentials and chat with him a few minutes to know that you could not be in better hands.

Hospital, Choosing a (Also see "Doctor, Choosing a," above)

Normally your choice of doctor dictates choice of hospital, since doctors practice only at certain ones. Still, two reasons for considering this a separate issue persist:

1. If you have no doctor, a plausible way of choosing one is to apply for one at a hospital chosen according to criteria we'll describe in a moment.

2. If your doctor stipulates a hospital that violates the standards we describe, you may want to consider a different hospital—and, maybe, doctor.

A large insurance company recently announced that policy holders needing a heart transplant (or kidney or liver transplant) must have it "at select hospitals it considers to have the best survival rates." All hospitals are not equal, not even close.

For instance, a 1988 survey of California hospitals that perform bypass surgery showed a range in death rates from 1.0% to 17.6%. The state median was 5.3%; but one expert maintained that for the usual mix of cases from easy to desperate, the bypass death rate should be no more than 3.5–4.0%.

Predictably, the high-mortality hospitals claimed that they somehow attract mostly tough cases. But an expert insisted that the patient mix was almost always the same. The significant difference was in number of operations performed. The survey highlighted "the lower death rates at hospitals that did many bypass surgeries compared to facilities that performed fewer surgeries." The chief of cardiac surgery at a hospital with one of the lowest death rates explained, "It is just like golf. If you don't practice your art every day, you are not going to be as slick." That goes for the entire surgical team.

One doctor commented, "The data imply that low-volume hospitals probably should not be doing heart surgery." No one can stop them; but you can refuse to let them practice on someone you love.

How can you tell? For bypass operations, the American College of Surgeons stipulates 150 a year. Yet among the lowest death rate hospitals in the survey, only one had fewer than *twice* that minimum. Ask your state medical association what minimum number they recommend for your procedure, and what its death rate is, statewide. Then ask the hospital what their numbers are. Another California survey revealed that *one-third* of the state's hospitals performed fewer than the recommended 150 minimum bypasses, which probably explains the 5.3% median when it should be 4.0% or less.

If your doctor insists on using a hospital that doesn't measure up, you certainly want to know why. It's hard to imagine an answer that could satisfy *us*. How about you?

Negotiating Fees

The survey about death rates cited above in "Hospital, Choosing a" revealed a wide range of hospital costs for bypass surgery: from about $16,000 at one hospital to an average of nearly $60,000 at another. Interestingly, the high-end hospital also had a high death rate. Hospitals generally do not negotiate fees, but you can shop around.

With doctors' fees it's different. Doctors are not given to haggling, but neither are their fees chiseled in marble. Judy Polk, who arranges finances for a group of them, says, "if physicians are approached openly and honestly upfront regarding any financial hardships—well, you know, physicians *help* people and they're not going to *not* help somebody they think they can help because of a money situation. I would say 99% of the doctors I've been working with over the last few years would make some sort of arrangement."

The words to ponder are "openly," "honestly," and "upfront." A doctor who prefers to remain anonymous (on the grounds that his family thinks he already does enough of this without actively courting more) says, "People who make it their business to find out who's the best and search them out are admirable—even if they can't pay. Some people will come in and say, 'I don't have a dime in my pocket, but I've heard that you're the best and I want you to do it.' I don't know of any expert who would turn down a patient like that."

CHAPTER 7

In the Hospital

Atmosphere and Attitude

I would like [the family] . . . to take as much of a positive attitude as possible about the future.

—Dr. Allan Lansing

Yes, you read it in the previous chapter. It's vital enough to memorize because it's central to the atmosphere you want to create for your patient and the attitude that leads to that atmosphere. The statement coincides with Dr. Lansing's assertion that the family must assume maximum responsibility for everything that will relieve the patient's anxieties over all issues extraneous to getting well.

Your attitude directly and measurably affects the patient. Polly Brown is clinical director at Dr. Lansing's hospital. As a practicing R.N., she saw it all the time. If a wife came in to visit, crying, she says, "I could see a difference on the monitor; the patient would start having PVCs. And you know that if the patient's upset, the heart works harder, the heart rate goes up, blood pressure can go up."

Less dramatic, though more pernicious, is the inevitable depersonalization of high-tech treatment that several doctors lamented in chapter 4. Since women generally fight dehumanization better than men, male family members (husbands of sick wives, especially) have to try more consciously.

What atmosphere and attitude can combat depersonalization? After bypass, patients must cough regularly to clear their lungs, although coughing hurts. To help, they hug a pillow to their chests. One California surgical group gives patients a teddy bear instead of a pillow. Its T-shirt identifies it as "Sir Koffalot," and proclaims, "A cough for your lungs/ a hug for your heart/ I'll help you to bear it/ by doing my part." Corny? Surely. Overly cute for some tastes? Maybe. But that's an example of the right spirit.

Beauty Shop Problems

Although the name comes from *Survive*, written particularly for wives of heart patients, this class of problems applies equally to men, indeed the whole family.

We called them "beauty shop" problems because one of the first manifestations for the wife of a patient involves agony over whether or not to go to a beauty shop before first visiting her husband. Any mirror tells her that the way she looks—haggard, bedraggled, red-eyed, and worried—may convince him that she assumes he's a goner. The obvious answer is a quick trip to the beauty shop for a rinse and set. It will certainly help physically and do wonders for morale.

Then comes the conflict. How can she even *think* of a beauty shop now! For *any* reason. In fact, what kind of monster must she be even to be having such a trivial, unworthy internal debate!

Unbidden thoughts like this can leave you a wreck—if you do not realize they are perfectly natural, shared in some form by nearly everyone in the same position. Notice that's *everyone*, man, woman, and child:

> *Mr. M:* And suddenly I realize what I'm thinking about is lunch and dinner out, but who's going to cook breakfast while she's in here? Susie's going to have her chest cut open and I'm worrying about omelets.

> *Mrs. D:* At first my feelings were hurt: I was on the outside, looking in. He was the star and I was just nobody. To get any attention around here you have to have a heart transplant.

> *Mrs. L:* Davie, the 12-year-old, was very upset and angry. That's how he responds to a crisis, he gets angry. "Well, what about fishing? And Daddy was going to do this with me and Daddy was going to do that."

You are not alone. Think your thoughts—and get on with what you have to do.

Children, What to Do with the

The problem obviously diminishes with children old enough to fend for themselves. But whether your children are young adults or toddlers, your arrangements for them should speak clearly of thought, planning, and above all consistency. This is a time of severe and mounting disruption in their lives, with overdoses of insecurity and inherent drama; children do not need the added uncertainty of wondering, day-to-day, who will look after them tomorrow.

The parent in the hospital shouldn't wonder either, particularly if that's the children's mother. You must relieve her mind, convince her that you've made plausible plans for somebody to deal with feeding, housekeeping, just *being* there for the children. She already feels guilty enough about leaving them to "indulge" herself in a heart condition.

Who should take care of your children?

Whoever you think most fond of them (and vice versa) and most regularly available. The likeliest candidates are, literally, the closest relatives—older brothers or sisters, of at least teen age. They can feel they are helping; the little ones will feel less strange about arrangements. One caution, though: the older ones must feel comfortable with the responsibility. Given that, it does not matter if normally the kids quarrel and scrap. This sense of pulling together and watching out for each other may do wonders for the relationship.

Next down the list are grandparents, aunts or uncles, or other close relatives—but close in affection and familiarity, not just blood. A friend of the family who has always known and loved the children is more suitable than a relative who hardly knows them.*

Have we overlooked a solution? Sending the children off somewhere to a nearby relative or friend if school is a problem, a camp or out-of-town relatives if not? After all, it's probably just for a short while. A trip might be a treat!

We have yet to meet a family that tried it without bitterly regretting the decision.

Mr. L, who had a heart attack while the whole family was away on vacation, could not travel home for several weeks. They talked it over and decided, says Mrs. L, to send the boys home for what seemed supremely logical reasons:

---

* Or, worse, dislikes them—a sentiment almost always requited.

Our youngest son was supposed to go to Cub Scout sleep-away camp, anyhow; our older son had lots of friends, and we thought he'd *like* staying with John's parents, who he's really close with. We wanted them to have as normal a routine as they could.

When we got home, we found them very, very upset. In fact, our youngest used to cry, "Why did you send us away?"

The older son had had a blowup with his grandmother because, for all the closeness, says Mrs. L, "she's not extremely sensitive to people's feelings and she certainly wasn't with him." He ended up staying at a friend's house.

Children resent being shuttled off and kept out of things. Keep them home, and consult them about any arrangements you propose to make for their care. A five-minute chat will demonstrate your concern for them and their needs. That's especially important for the older ones, but applies to children of any age. Even if, in fact, special arrangements are unnecessary, they'll feel better knowing you have considered the problem. As Dr. Kent Trinkle says, "Children are usually much stronger and more perceptive than we tend to give them credit for." Giving them a chance to assure you that "you mustn't worry" about them is a considerable service to their self-image just now. It's one positive way they can feel they're helping.

Denial, Problem of

"Denial" is the term doctors use to describe a reaction to serious illness that's so common they almost expect it. The authors of a psychiatric study of 50 heart patients at Massachusetts General Hospital wrote this:

> The defense mechanism of denial is defined as the conscious or unconscious repudiation of part or all of the total available meaning of an event to allay fear, anxiety, or other unpleasant effects. The term "major denial" is used to describe patients who stated unequivocally that they felt no fear at any time throughout their hospital stay; 20 out of 50 examined were in this group. . .

Two out of five simply ignored the fact that they had a potentially fatal condition. The doctors also said that another 20 patients evidenced "partial denial."

No one is immune. One doctor, himself a heart attack patient, says:

> I was amazed at my own reaction. I see denial in patients all the time; it's one of the things I know I must always be on the lookout for in my patients.

And, suddenly there I am, denying to myself that I've "really had a heart attack." I knew what I was doing and how silly it was, but I couldn't help myself!

What difference does it make? "Patients with denial," says Dr. John Strobeck, "may not want to deal with the specifics of their condition. They want to hear that, 'It wasn't so bad.' Or, 'This doesn't mean that you have to give up this or that.'" They may turn doctors' instructions into a game of, Let's see what we can get away with without the doctor finding out. Trouble is, doctors do not play; they just keep score. And this is a game in which, sooner or later, everybody knows the score.

Denial by the family is only slightly less common. It starts with some variation on the theme of this wife's first reaction when told that her husband had suffered a heart attack at the office: "I couldn't believe it! I thought, 'Well, there just has to be a mistake. I just spoke to him a couple of hours ago on the phone!'" The transition from, "I can't believe it" to, "somehow it isn't *really* true" is as easy as it is pernicious.

You surely don't suffer what the psychiatrists called "major denial" (you'd scarcely be reading this if "nothing really happened"). But you must purge yourself of any lingering doubts about severity because you must make sure the patient does not harbor the least doubt. If you aren't sure, insist that a doctor intervene.

Doctors and Nurses, How to Talk with (Also see "Help and Information, Why You Need and Where to Get," below)

You'll find all the reasons you and the patient need information in "Help and Information," below. Part of the family's role in relieving the patient's mind is to make sure the necessary questions are asked and answered. The family should, as Dr. DeVries puts it, "act as the patient's ombudsman with the medical profession, go out and gather information on behalf of the patient."

That isn't always easy. It's hard *not* to be "intimidated by the professionals"*: they're so visibly busy; they may seem aloof. In any case, as one nurse acknowledged, "medical schools don't teach communication." For every doctor like Humana's Allan Lansing, who makes a policy of simplifying things and using understandable analogies, many use jargon as hard to decipher as their handwriting. Nurses tend to be a little more practiced in dealing with people.

---

* See "Doctors, Referrals from and to" in chapter 6.

In any case, your job is to insist on understandable answers. Now, insistence doesn't mean impertinence or impoliteness. You'll get the best results by being patently considerate of professionals' time and energy. Start by appointing one person to speak for the entire family and friends. "That way," says Dr. Sam Teichman, "the doctor explains it once, not eight times, and feels that family is acting responsibly."

The next step is to write down everyone's questions. As Mrs. B explains the need,

> I had a lot of questions. Why does Dan have to stay on this medication for 60 days but that one for a year? Is it better to walk as many miles as you can, or a fast pace for a certain number of miles? Can he play tennis? When?
>
> I had at least 10 questions, and if I didn't write them down I'd draw as blank as soon as I looked at the doctor.

You won't get all that many answer sessions with doctors or nurses; be ready with a list. And be ready to accommodate their schedules— especially the doctors'. Dr. Teichman provides a suitable family member monologue:

> If you haven't got time right now to sit down and answer the 27 questions I've collected from the whole family, let me know when it's convenient for you. But please do make time—because these questions are important to us. Or point me to somebody who can give me most of the answers—and I'll be back to you with the rest.

Between them, says Dr. Teichman, a resident and head nurse can likely dispatch, say, 22 of the questions, leaving only five for the harder-pressed doctor.

Finally, whenever possible, ask your questions in your patient's presence. This is not a contest to see who can gain, and use, information for purposes of control. Kim Wimsatt, a clinical coordinator at Humana, cringes whenever a family member wants to talk with her "out in the hallway." She knows what's coming:

> The wife will say, "He likes to go bowling; he can't do that now, can he?" Or, "You do know that he smokes." Or, "He eats a gallon of ice cream a night."
>
> She knows if she said it in the room, he'd be ready to climb up off the bed and choke her or rebut what she's saying.

To counter this, Wimsatt conscientiously includes both. "I try," she says, "to let them know it's going to be a team effort." Following the necessary prescriptions and proscriptions must be a team effort, and unless the patient is firmly on the team, your side cannot win.

Going Home, Getting Ready for

The patient and all relevant family members must be clear on diet and on exercise and activity.

In the more up-to-date hospitals, you won't need this section. Various staff experts shower you with the information you need before going home. At others, you have to make your own arrangements. The problem is that you have little time to get started, thanks to today's comparatively short hospital stays, because most of what you should do is best done at the hospital.

First, diet. Of course if the doctor specifies a diet, that's it. More likely, if the doctor mentions the subject, it will be in platitudes about "eating sensibly" and "cutting down fats." You need particulars. And, as one doctor ruefully admits, "the doctor is not usually the best place to start." Instead, if the hospital has a staff dietitian, ask for an appointment. Failing that, ask for a reference to any registered dietitian nearby. If the hospital declines references,* try the Yellow Pages, or write or phone the American Dietetic Association, 216 W. Jackson Blvd., Chicago, IL 60606-6995 (312) 899-0040. Note that you want a *registered* dietitian, not just someone who sets up as a nutrition expert. If in doubt, check with the ADA. See chapter 10 for the specifics of what you want to discuss, and also for the names of useful books and pamphlets.

Your next concern is activity and exercises. Except in unusual cases, patients today start exercising while in the hospital, and should go home with a clear program for continued exercise and a clear idea of what they can do and when they can do it. Chapter 11 provides a complete rundown. If your hospital does not offer a formal rehabilitation program, arrange for your own now. Try to locate an established rehabilitation program nearby that your patient can join; the psychological assurance of exercise monitoring, alone, makes it worth the price.

In any case, you must start with an outline by the doctor *in the patient's presence* of how much and what kind of exercise and what kind of activity is allowed and when it is allowed. Demand specifics.

Help and Information, Why You Need and Where to Get

First, you should recognize the need for certain information. Studies show that patients who are more knowledgeable about their

---

* It's certainly beginning to sound as though you're tied up with the wrong hospital.

condition, who understand what's being done and should be done, generally experience shorter hospital stays and quicker overall recoveries. Dr. William DeVries gives us an elemental example of how it works: Everyone's been saying the bypass was a rousing success, but a day or so later the patient feels weak, nauseated, rotten. That makes the patient apprehensive: is there something *they're not telling*? "A doctor can take care of that very rapidly," says Dr. DeVries. "You just tell the patient, 'Don't worry, it's natural to feel that way; everybody feels rotten and weak after surgery.'" Mind relieved, the patient can concentrate on getting well.

Simple. But many doctors may just zip in, glance at the EKG, see everything's OK, say, "You're doing fine," and whiz out. Someone has to make sure the patient gets the information that will make the difference.

Once recovered and back home, the patient will likely have to make some life adjustments. "The adjustments," says Dr. Shahbudin Rahimtoola, "can only come with a knowledge of what the disease is, what the prognosis, extent of damage, and what limitations all that calls for, what the outcome is likely to be."

As far as practicable, everyone should get the same information at the same time. Besides the reasons discussed on page 87, health care professionals have noticed after the trauma of surgery or heart attack many patients forget part or all of what they're told during the hospital stay. Moreover, the family needs maximum information in order to be of maximum use. "Once they understand all of this," says Dr. Zahi Masri, "they can be of tremendous help to the patient, to the doctor, to the nursing staff. To everybody."

You also probably need the information for your own psychological well-being. Mrs. C states the case with self-insight and honesty:

> When we met with the doctor for the first time, he was wonderful.
> At first, Joe didn't want me to come in; he doesn't deal with medical things very well. And I was sitting out there in the waiting room—and I was starting to get nervous. I felt really shut out, and I felt like I wanted to know.
> So I knocked and I said, "Can I please come in?" I said, "I really need to come in." Because I was a wreck.

Obviously, the best source for the needed information is doctors, nurses, and other health care professionals. Your access to these people is best while your patient remains in the hospital, a period that continues to shrink as hospital stays typically grow shorter. To borrow a word from the wife of one former patient, you have to be "tenacious."

Helpless and Alone, Feeling

Well of course you feel that way. Of all those we've talked with, only one says, "I never felt alone." She says it was not religion, just the love and respect of family, children and friends. Maybe so; more likely it was confusion over the meaning of "alone." The more typical feeling—including among those who profess deep religion, and felt sustained by it—was expressed by a woman who says,

Oh! you are by yourself! Friends come and sit and try to tell you everything's going to be all right; but they don't *know*. . . .

You're alone because no one seems to understand the problems you face; the sympathy of the most well-meaning is not informed, so it really doesn't comfort or do justice to the problem.

As for a feeling of helplessness, someone you love is an island of need entirely surrounded by competent professionals doing the one thing you would like to do and can't, something specific and of substance to help.

What can you do about these feelings?

The essential message of this book is that others have had the same feelings and problems, are sharing them with you, sharing the things that helped them, including the mistakes they made—all in an effort to keep you from repeating them. You are not alone.

You *are* helpless in the sense of not being of any specific medical use.* Even if you happen to be a doctor or nurse, *this* case is in someone else's hands.

Still you have a distinct role, not just for the long term; immediately, still in the hospital. One concrete example comes from an R.N.:

The hardest thing is not to have an active role. I tell the patient's wife, especially if he's going for a cath, an angioplasty, "Yes, ma'am, you can do something for me: please hold his hand; please be with him and be as calm as you can be. And reassure him."

In the larger sense, everything we talk about in this chapter is of help, directly and medically. That's *why*, as we've seen, doctors insist that the hardest patient to deal with is one without a family.

If you truly are helpless and truly aren't helping, shame!

How the Patient Is

You need consider only two facts on this subject, equally true and important, although seemingly contradictory.

---

* For a vital exception, see "You as Authority," below.

Remember from chapter 4 that, possibly excepting valve surgery, no procedure or treatment ever cures a heart condition,* only palliates it. As one doctor told a patient after bypass surgery, "Your heart now is as good as it was when you were 18; but the rest of your body is still 55—plus your blood vessels are badly corroded." He probably added that those bypasses weren't going to keep their adolescent patency unless their owner took better care of them than he had the originals. That, of course, is the point of emphasizing the absence of cures in this field.

Still, remember even as you read the next section, and when you see the patient, that the procedure or the treatment *has* palliated the problem. The heart *has*, at one surgical or procedural or medicinal stroke, become much better than it was before, and many if not all of the symptoms that made life hell will have disappeared once the patient is over the trauma of treatment (or infarction) that's making him or her *look* the way they do. Give it time.

How the Patient Looks

In 1974 a woman remembered her first glimpse of her husband in an intensive care unit:

> I didn't realize what was going to happen ahead of time. What I'd be seeing. . . I just went right in.
> It was the scariest thing I ever saw.
> I looked at him, then I looked around and saw other patients and some looked like—well suddenly I couldn't stand it. I just ran out of there, tears falling out of my eyes.
> It was very frightening!

Today's surgical and coronary care techniques make those of that era seem primitive. So how does the patient look today? A sampling:

> *Mrs. K:* They warned me, but nothing they say can prepare you for it, no way.

> *Clinical Coordinator:* . . . a shocking experience, to say the least.

> *Mrs. S:* The terrible thing was the intensive care. I had seen it before, but this was someone else; it wasn't my husband. And when I saw him connected to all of those tubes it was frightening.

---

* If someone argues that transplant for cardiomyopathy gets rid of a condition that almost surely cannot return, and so constitutes a cure, we surrender; except that a transplant, however mercifully life-giving, is scarcely our notion of a cure. And you've surely gathered that we bow to none in enthusiasm for the operation.

Mrs. W: It was frightening to see those machines and tubes in the ICU—and the *look* in Dad's eyes: like a wounded animal; teary, glassy, yet moving all over. . .

Mr. F: Right after surgery, her face was swollen, tongue hanging out, tubes in. I said to the doctor, "Isn't she *gorgeous!*" And I'm thinking, "Doesn't she look terrible, and uncomfortable."

Dr. Julian Frieden, himself a surgeon, couldn't sleep after seeing his wife after her bypass surgery.

Nothing has changed. For all the progress in treatment, a heart attack or coronary surgery hits you like that 10-ton truck, and the body reacts.

Strangely enough, Mr. F's "Isn't she gorgeous" was on the mark. He said it because his wife was *alive* and was, from the moment the operation ended, on the way back to a real life after years of languishing. The tubes, the pallor, the haunted look—even the evident discomfort—none of it means anything; indeed, most patients cannot even recall the first day or so. What means everything is the look you *will* see soon. And that is gorgeous.

Length of Stay

We can say this for certain, it's shorter. Shorter for surgery and heart attack than when we wrote *Survive*, shorter every time you survey the subject. Miss B went with her father to UCLA for an angiogram—to take him home a few hours later; insurance did not cover *any* hospital stay for that. At Dr. John Hutchinson's hospital in New Jersey they no longer have time to give patients and families a preoperative educational visit to intensive care; insurance coverage mandates admission only the night before, not two days before an operation as it used to be.

How about after an operation? "We used to have everybody in the hospital 10 to 12 days after open heart surgery," says Dr. Allan Lansing in Kentucky. "Then it got down to 9 to 10; now it's frequently—well, I operated on my brother-in-law a week ago, an aortic valve replacement, and he was out of the hospital in six days." That was unusual, but by no means unexampled. Across the country it's the same.

For reasonably routine heart attacks the stay was once two to five days in a Coronary Care Unit, four to six weeks in the hospital. Today, says Dr. Sam Teichman, in San Francisco, CCU stays more often measure 24 to 48 *hours*, with the patient sometimes back to work in a few weeks.* Particularly aggressive cardiologists may send patients home the third day; most will have evaluated patients during exercise on a stationary bike or treadmill as early as the fifth day. Home on the fifth day is not uncommon. (But neither, please note, is a two-week stay; be *sure* to read the section below!) "The trend is clear," says Dr. Teichman, "If they're safely sending them home on day three in Michigan, the guys in Mississippi can safely shorten hospital stay from nine to seven or eight to six." Today's patients do not dawdle in bed.

Length of Stay, Comparing Notes on

Don't.

No good can come of it. If you're cheered to learn that your patient is going home a day sooner than Al, you'll be that much more worried to learn that it's two days later than Zelma, and you can torture yourself up and down the rest of the alphabet. None of it means anything. Different doctors follow different practices in the matter; different patients need different treatment, and the different treatment may bear not the slightest relationship to "how well they're doing."

When we gave this same advice in *Survive*, we noted that no one had ever taken it. What's changed? Only that comparisons then might be a matter of weeks; now it's days. We expect that someday families will agonize over the discovery that patient X, who came in at the same time, yesterday, is going home at 11 this morning, while *their* patient has to languish until 3 *p.m.* What can it mean? Is the doctor keeping something from us? Are there . . . problems?

Don't.

Nurses, Cultivation of

Polly Brown practiced as a nurse for years; now she directs the clinical coordinators at Humana in Louisville. She says,

> I'd hate being a patient in many hospitals. There's no privacy. No one knocks on your door. There's no . . . respect.
>
> You get an 18-year-old saying to Mr. Jones, who is 70: "Come on, Joe!" That's not treating someone with respect. If patients feel better being called by their first name, they're the ones who should tell you that.

---

* In 1988, the Chicago Bears football coach, Mike Ditka, suffered a heart attack, was treated with the clot-dissolver, TPA, and was back on the sidelines coaching his team on a Sunday 12 days later.

> You can humanize the experience by being polite, showing respect, by knocking on doors—and if I ever see a nurse not knock on doors, she's gonna hear from me, and they all know it, because I can't *stand* it!

It works both ways. A nurse who deals mostly with transplant recipients reported how emotionally exhausting that can be: she becomes so rapt by their progress, so frustrated if they don't seem to be trying to get well, especially when some patients and their families prove unreasonably demanding and querulous, even mean. She must make an additional emotional effort not to retaliate, to keep reminding herself that, after all, the patients are unwell, the families distraught.

She shouldn't have to, especially in regard to families. Your tension, or even anxiety and distress, really bears no relation to how you deal with nurses. Just remember that although in the course of their duties they sometimes perform the messiest, most menial tasks, they are professionals, highly trained and, today, highly paid.

You have every right to expect, even demand, close attention and care for your patient; you should require answers to your questions. But, equally, you must ask for things with courtesy, respect, and consideration, realizing that these people are generally rushed and worked to frazzles. You do not in any way offend by reminding them whenever they forget some aspect of care or some request; as one nurse puts it, "Those kinds of things I *appreciate* because I probably get 150 of them a day, and if someone reminds me when I forget, you aren't 'bothering' me, you're helping me do my job." *How* you ask and *how* you remind are another matter.

Chances are, no matter what you do, the nurses will take excellent care of your patient. Still, it's only human to do that little extra for people you like. So even if someone could prove it didn't matter, we would still go out of our way to make friends of the nurses, to engage their sympathy and interest on behalf of the person we love who's in their care.

The best way to do it is whatever comes most naturally. After all, you are expressing genuine appreciation and friendliness for people doing something that's important to you.

Here is how one wife handled it:

> I introduced myself to the nurses, and I told them all, "This is a very dear, sweet, special human being and we are madly in love with each other, and I want you to give him extra special care." And I went into the gift shop, and I brought back a bunch of cookies and candy, and I said, "Just to remind you how sweet *he* is!"

Her attitude, demonstrated and expressed, was calculated to make the nurses care about the couple and about the patient.

It makes a valuable point about gifts. Money is generally inappropriate (except, of course, with a private nurse); but *things* are fine. They *should not* be expensive; you are not tendering a bribe or tip, just an expression of gratitude. If you give things you've made, a cake, cookies, fudge, all the better; but stuff from the gift shop is fine, too. Understand, gifts are not mandatory; these men and women are taking care of patients, not holding them for ransom. If giving gifts feels right, do it.

In any case, you can make nurses care about you (and by extension the patient) by evidencing an interest in them as people. That shouldn't be hard; nurses tend to be interesting people.

Psychological Reaction, the Patient's

> Having a heart attack. . . something striking at what is perceived as the core of your existence. . . can affect a person psychologically much more than anything else. . .
>
> Some don't react right away; maybe denial prevents them from reacting. But when they begin to deal with it, and begin to react. . . it's very confusing to the family.
>
> —Dr. John Strobeck

That applies to nearly any heart condition for the central reason that the underlying problem will never go away.

The first result is a sudden, demoralizing intimation of mortality. "Frequently," says Dr. Shahbudin Rahimtoola, "that's the first time the individual has really faced up to the fact of being mortal." We all "know" we're going to die—some day. A heart condition serious enough to put someone in the hospital, says Dr. Rahimtoola,

> . . . brings this feeling that it's not open-ended. The person thinks a lot more about death, and often makes statements about death which the family doesn't understand. They tend sometimes to pooh pooh it; but they've got to realize that this individual sees an end to life and it enters the psyche much more.

Even the reasonable assurance that death is not imminent may not help. Few patients can help thinking, "Yes, but what kind of life will it be? What will I have to give up? Smoking surely. Drinking? The foods I like? Sports? Activities? Social life? And how about sex? What will this mean to that part of life?" Suddenly patients can easily start to apprehend the possibility of life without zest or flavor.

How about work? Career goals, plans, dreams, can suddenly seem ashes. Even without fear of losing a job,* patients often assume that people with demonstrated heart problems are no longer desirable employees. What can they do? Promise never to have another heart attack, never let the bypasses clog up?

At this point, patients routinely ask the same basic question. Why me? Why not someone else? (Names furnished on request.)

Pam Moore, nurse-manager of the rehabilitation center at Brotman Memorial Hospital in Los Angeles, says, "You can analyze it until you're blue in the face and not find adequate answers to their question. Men seem to have this problem more than women because they want to pick it apart and have a *reason* behind everything." All anyone can do, she says, is accept the fact and get on with living. But that's not much comfort, so patients (particularly men) typically react in three other ways.

First, there's the denial we examined above.

Second, some men compensate in the area of sex. With such dramatically shorter hospital stays, the locale of this reaction may shift from hospital to home, but the principle remains the same. It constitutes what we called in *Survive* "The Grand Turk" reactions, so wildly unexpected, so unlike the patient, they can be more troublesome than later, actual sexual readjustments. For example, Mr. L had suffered a heart attack five weeks before, and for the past two weeks had been exhibiting most distressing behavior. Physically he was fine; the doctor said he could go home the next week (this was in 1973). In his early 40s, Mr. L was normally a very dignified, quiet, and considerate person. But now, his wife told us, he had turned into a dirty old man, leering at nurses, patting, pinching, his "conversation" a monologue of dirty jokes relieved only by suggestive remarks. At one point their teenage daughter left the room in tears and shock.

In the course of a distraught hour-and-a-half phone call, we assured Mrs. L that The Grand Turk Syndrome was, if not routine, at least not rare. More important, it runs its course in a matter of weeks. Patients generally don't even remember feeling that way. Sure enough, once back home, Mr. L soon stoutly denied he ever had said or done any such things or ever would or could.

---

* Not necessarily an irrational fear. Mr. G had been a full-time consultant, travelling to the clients of a California company on a schedule whose brutal demands Mrs. G is sure brought on his heart attack. While Mr. G was recuperating, the boss called to ask, "When can we have your office?" Soon, UPS delivered seven boxes of his personal office effects. "What kind of people are these?" Mrs. G asks. The answer is, fortunately, "reasonably rare."

The third reaction is hostility—usually turned on the patient's spouse. This more commonly afflicts male patients, but not overwhelmingly so. As Polly Brown explains the mechanism, people who have always been forceful, even dominant (the perfect heart attack type), suddenly find themselves helpless, with those sudden thoughts of mortality. "So now," says Brown, "he is going to be very bitter; he's also going to be very short-tempered; he's almost going to try to pick a quarrel in order to take the upper hand again, and the wife doesn't understand that." Neither, if it's turned around, does the husband, or the children, or anyone else in the family.

Except that now you do, which points the way for what to do about all three psychological reactions.

First, help your patient understand that, inevitable intimations of mortality aside, life probably will not be so different. As Dr. Strobeck says,

> The bulk of patients will be able to return to doing exactly what they were doing before. They just have to be smarter about it.
> Look at what it is in the overall life style of the patient that predisposes to heart attack, and invariably those elements can be modified. *Quantity* must be modified; the *quality* can remain the same.

Beyond that, just realize that all this is normal and temporary. We once asked a wife if it would have helped at the time to know beforehand the reasons for her husband's seemingly inexplicable hostility. "Ohhh. . . *yes!*" she said. "As Dr. Spock says, *this* is typical of age eighteen months, *this* is typical of two years. If someone had said, *this* is typical of a heart attack, I could have taken. . . *anything!*"

Now you know.

Social Life, Your

Given today's short hospital stays, this issue probably won't arise. Not that it's unimportant. If it comes up during the hospital stay, see the same entry in chapter 8.

Surgery, Your Rights During

This one's easy: you have a right to know what's going on. Good hospitals won't compel you to assert that right. The surgical teams will have someone—generally a nurse, often titled "clinical coordinator"—whose specific job is to keep the family informed during each major stage of the operation. They generally also help educate the patient and family beforehand, and see that the patient and family meet with the right rehabilitation and education specialists after the operation. Typically, coordinators do a marvelous job. Mrs. N remembers the night of her husband's transplant, a time of understandably unbearable tension:

> Nancy was there, fortunately, and every couple of hours she would come down and tell me what was going on. Fill us in, take us step-by-step through the procedure. She was just a doll! Wonderful lady.

Not all hospitals provide the service. And even at the best of them, things can go wrong. "You have to be assertive," says Miss P, who tells a horror story about when her father had his bypass at the *same* hospital as Mrs. N's husband!

The operation, scheduled for 11 a.m., was postponed until five that afternoon, but no one told the family, huddled in the cavernous lobby, until well after the time they had concluded that something must be terribly wrong to be taking that long. The coordinator had introduced herself the night before, but didn't seem to be around. The family felt her absence most sorely that evening when the thought struck that since the group's senior surgeon was an Orthodox Jew, and this was Friday, would he simply stop operating at sundown? Surely not, but. . .

They needed questions answered and could find no one. Miss P's sister says,

> I was ready to go into the operating room and find out what was going on; we were at that stage. "Why isn't there anyone to tell us? All these people who made promises; they aren't doing it."

The answer, the aggrieved sisters agree—and it obviously applies to hospitals without designated coordinators—is to demand the name, phone, and office number of someone who will be responsible for answering your questions during the operation. Then, if they don't follow through, as Miss P says, "be assertive."

Visiting

Like some others, this issue fades in importance as hospital stays shorten. Yet that very shortness can create pitfalls. When you reckoned the average stay in weeks, not days, friends and relatives had plenty of time to "pay their respects," to show the patient their love and concern by visiting *during the hospital stay*, a visit somehow charged with more meaning than those at home. With that window now usually so narrow, you must guard against excess, both in number and duration.

Mr. C arranges music for a large band. He was 75 and still active when he had a complicated, lengthy bypass operation* that kept him on the operating table six hours. The draining nature of the surgery combined with his age to make visits unwise, especially since his profession and popularity meant that people wanting to see him thronged the corridor. Mrs. C simply refused to let visitors in the room. She talked to them at length when she could; when too tired, she simply explained that George was not allowed visitors, but that she'd of course tell him they came. It was, she says, her hardest chore, being diplomatic on her husband's behalf. But she felt not the least guilt about saying no.

Mrs. J's husband was allowed visitors, but some created a problem. At first, she says, she didn't handle it well:

> If you have company too long, they will tire you so much you can relapse. It happened to Don in the hospital. Two guys from the office stayed an hour. Don was exhausted, plus the fact they were discussing business, three days after his surgery. I couldn't get a word in edgewise to get these young men out of here.

The nurse told her what to do: "Valerie said, 'You're going to have to be rude, and if people's feelings are hurt, they'll have to be hurt.'" If you explain the situation pleasantly, and their feelings are still hurt, what kind of friends are they?

Miss P and her family encountered another common problem after surgery (see "Surgery," above). Her father really didn't feel like seeing anyone except the immediate family. They displayed the exact right attitude:

> Fortunately most people are smart enough to ask. We didn't hurt any feelings—but, frankly, I wouldn't have cared. My father's health was more important and so were his wishes.
>
> If people get their feelings hurt because they can't understand why people might not want company after heart surgery, that's *their* problem. But people generally were nice enough about it. They all wanted to be called and told how everything went; the phone outside the waiting room became our personal phone.

Weaning Anxiety

The name comes from the *New England Journal of Medicine*, whose study showed that 25% of patients own up to nervousness over

---

* Preceded by an endarterectomy, where they open a major artery to cut away what's clogging it.

leaving a special care unit for a regular room.* In *Survive*, we reported that a nurse put the figure closer to 90%, relying not on what patients said (as the *Journal* did) but what she observed.

We imagined this another dead (or highly moribund) issue. Today's stays in CCU or ICU, we assumed, are normally too short to engender the sense of fragility in a patient that would result in anxiety over being "unplugged." But Polly Brown assures us that weaning anxiety persists, and that it can also affect the spouse if not the entire family. She points out that most everyone gets through the crisis of special care well enough, especially given the medical cosseting each patient receives. But then, when it's time to leave, she says,

> . . . your umbilical cord's cut. The nurse isn't always there. The patient's frightened when he maybe doesn't get pain medicine as quickly if he has pain. It looks like you're forgotten, thrown out into the real world.
>
> And no matter how much explaining you do, the wife gets even more anxious. She'll ask you, "Should I stay in the hospital all the time? I'm afraid to leave the room."

The answer remains the same. No patient leaves CCU or ICU until that degree of supervision is superfluous. The response of nurses (with pain medication, for instance) is not as instant because the need is not as critical. The monitoring continues; in the unlikelihood of an emergency, the monitor will let the professionals know a lot sooner than either spouse *or* patient can tell by observation.

Weaning anxiety isn't a dead letter in the hospital; but it should be.

Who Should Be Told?

There is no blanket answer except, "It all depends." Indeed, you probably do best to turn the question around and think of it as, Who *shouldn't* be told. List everyone you instinctively feel should be told, then ask yourself about each: Is there any reason this one should not know, at least right now? What possible bad consequences could flow?

Obvious examples spring to mind. Examine them by categories.

Parents

One wife decided not to tell her husband's mother that he'd just suffered a heart attack because she feared the shock might kill her. The elderly, bedridden woman had suffered several heart attacks herself. Even that decision was not automatic. She weighed the

---

* See "Weaning Anxiety, More" in chapter 8 for the related problem at home.

chance of her mother-in-law's finding out from other sources. That shock, she realized, would be worse than if it came from her or the old woman's other son. When she concluded there was small chance, she decided to wait until she could start the report by stating absolutely that the woman's son was all right. "Then," says the wife, "she would be told with the proper people in attendance, her doctor, and so on."

Another wife decided to wait until her husband was out of the hospital and clearly on the mend to tell her mother-in-law, an excitable, nervous woman with an advanced talent for setting everyone on edge, with her son heading the list. Fortunately, she lived on the opposite coast and would be unlikely to hear the news immediately. "As his mother," the wife says,

> she had a right to know. But. . . the most important thing was for my husband to get well. And for me to *stay* well, to help make him well.
>
> Having his mother there would have been difficult for him—and impossible for me. She would have gone to pieces, and it just would have brought me down.

You can always explain, later, that you didn't want to worry them unduly, or you wanted to spare them a trip. You can even tell the truth. In any case, if you consider your decision carefully, you will be armed with the assurance of having done what you thought right.

Children

Even with them, it's not an automatic decision, even if they're adults. Mrs. C, wife of the music arranger (see "Visiting," above), decided not to tell his daughter from a previous marriage "until after the surgery, until George was home and mending." The girl had never accepted Mrs. C, had always quarreled with her father, who was rather relieved when she moved across the country. If she flew back for the operation, Mrs. C says, "it would make more problems in the family, more trauma; and we just didn't need more emotional upheaval." His son, on the other hand, lived close by, was always supportive, and of course was told.

All three sons of Mrs. N knew their father would receive a transplant. But Mrs. N decided to summon only their eldest son, Sam, to the hospital that night. He's technical minded, fascinated by the process, and calm. Bob is artistic, a musician, rather squeamish; he worked nights at a TV station, and his mother insisted he *not* come to the hospital, although she did call him at work to relay the coordinator's progress reports. Cal, "young and naive," also worked nights; his mother decided not to let him know even that the operation was on until next morning when she could report it a success. "I didn't want to scare him," she says.

When you tell younger ones is less important than what you tell them. Even for the youngest, whatever variation of "sick" you choose in order to account for the hospital stay (e.g., "very, very sick," "sick in a grown-up way") will almost surely lead to, "Is Daddy (or Mommy) going to die?"

"You can't tell a child absolutes," insists a nurse who regularly talks with many parents faced with the problem. "You can't make a promise like, 'Absolutely not!'"

"What if something does happen?" agrees Mrs. A, whose 9-year-old asked the question. "I said, I don't think so, but he's really sick and the doctors are giving him medicine, and he has to stay in the hospital and rest so he can get better."

We can't think of a better answer.

Whatever you tell the children, by all means tell their favorite teacher or the principal of their school. If they are not yet in school, make sure whoever is with them knows. It will explain why they may be acting a little strangely.

Business Associates

With company insurance or state disability involved, you have no choice about informing employers. But *when* to tell may be another matter. Today's shorter hospital stays give you leeway—in case, like Mrs. J in "Visiting," above, you fear taxing hospital visits.

It probably won't matter. Despite the truly disgraceful reaction of Mr. G's employer, recounted above in "Psychological Reaction," observers generally agree that people today are more understanding about heart conditions.

Even so, especially if the patient is a professional or entrepreneur, there's no rush to tell most clients, customers, associates, employees, or competitors. Certainly the matter of whom and what to tell needs ventilation with the patient beforehand. You can always tell people something tomorrow; you will find it harder to make them forget tomorrow what you blabbed today.

The same goes for any of your own business associates, this time including employer, unless it's *your* insurance that foots the bills.

The best test is probably the same as for state secrets: a "need to know" basis.

You as Authority

While contemplating your isolation and lamenting your inability to render substantive help (see "Alone and Helpless," above), remember the one kind of direct, medical help you and the entire family can give health professionals. You can warn them if something is wrong with the patient that they might not pick up nearly as quickly as you can.

We wrote in "Weaning," above, that the monitor does it faster, but that's heart-connected emergencies. Other things can go wrong slowly, building chronically, whose signs are subtle changes in the patient's attitude, personality, or behavior. You are the authority in that area. Indeed, the health professionals might never notice.

We touched on the subject in chapter 5, "Transplants," where it's vital because patients often must wait long periods at home, dosed with powerful medications, and, after surgery, live with powerful medication as a constant companion. With other heart treatments instances are less common. But you must be on the lookout.

One example will give you the idea.

Mr. K had a heart attack eight years ago, and Mrs. K became convinced that he was not rallying as he should be. "I knew the doctors were competent," she says, "but a lot had to do with my knowledge of Bob's personality and reactions." The doctors had prescribed Valium, the tranquilizer, to help him relax. To Mrs. K, he seemed almost torpid. She knew he reacted strongly to medication, and almost never took any. "We had a long discussion with the doctor," Mrs. K says,

> . . . or, actually, I did; Bob was really out of it, in another world. The doctor said, "Well, that's a result of his condition." But I felt it wasn't: that wasn't his personality; he's a fighter, and he wasn't fighting. So I said, "Take him off the Valium. What can happen?"
>
> His reaction just didn't seem normal. But how would the doctor know?

Was it extraordinary to speak up? When a doctor prescribes, who are we to say different?

Mrs. K didn't think it unusual. She says,

> I wouldn't have said, "Shouldn't he be on one heart medicine rather than something else?" I'm not knowledgeable at all. But I did know his psyche and his spirit, and I had seen him in other circumstances.
>
> And if the doctor had felt that I was off the wall, and it was life-threatening, he would have said no. But this medication was given for psychological reasons, and I could tell it was having the wrong effect.
>
> They tried taking him off, and he began to become interested, and once he became interested, he started to recover much quicker.

You may not know, as in this case, exactly what is making the difference; but if you spot one, be sure to speak up. The professionals don't resent it; they count on it.

CHAPTER 8

At Home

Actually, the focus of the rest of the book is on what happens "at home." This chapter examines the "recuperation" period—until, for instance, return to work, or until doctors' appointments become infrequent, routine checkups.

Atmosphere and Your Attitude

A home is not a hospital; avoid turning yours into even the suggestion of one. If the health professionals thought your patient* still needed a hospital, your patient would still be in the hospital. They know you and the rest of the family are not doctors or nurses, much less heart monitors; they would not send into your hands any patient who still needed those people and things standing by.

Logic is one thing, emotion another. Nearly all family members experience anxious moments. In 1973 one wife told us,

> The first week he is home you wake up at all hours—five, six times, every night. And, you know, just look at him. Like, is he still . . . breathing?

---

* A *most* inappropriate word from here on. But we beg your indulgence and understanding of why we must continue to use it: we can't think of any other. In fact no single word describes what we mean, i.e., your *husband/wife/mother/father/grandparent/brother/ sister/"significant other"/whatever-who-was-a-patient-but-is-now-recovering/recovered- yet-still-has-the-underlying-condition-because-heart-treatment-is-palliative-not-curative- so-must-change-lifestyle-in-certain-ways.* So "patient," however inappropriate, it remains—which at least serves to remind that the lifestyle changes are for keeps.

Today, a wife says,

I'd just check from time to time to see he's OK. See that those
bedclothes are coming up and down.

In fact, they might not be; in deep sleep, normal breathing is often too
shallow to detect easily—something to keep in mind. If you *must* do
something, hold a mirror or feather to the nostrils. You may feel silly,
but it beats waking the person—the way hospitals do, sometimes, in
order to administer sleeping pills. Your home is *not* a hospital.

You should, however, take certain precautions. They're most
important if the patient suffered a heart attack, but are sensible for
any home.

Cardiopulmonary Resuscitation

Everyone should know CPR anyway. It's easy and quick to learn.
Call your local "Y" or the Red Cross or Heart Association or Police
or Fire Department to locate the nearest classes. Merely learning constitutes a positive step because it instills in everyone, patient included,
confidence that all are equipped for emergencies (and care enough to
become so).

Emergencies

Find out where to call for the fastest help—usually the paramedics—
then paste a label with the name and number on each phone in your
home. Include your address, including apartment number. Point it
out to everyone, especially children. Often the number is "911." If the
"number" is "0" for operator, specify what the caller should do and
say. That label might look like this:

EMERGENCY—Dial "Operator" and say:
"Fire Department Rescue Squad"
"Address with apartment number"

You might also give the doctor's number, but that's all. In emergencies
people are, by definition, rushed, excited, and frightened. So keep it
simple. And notice the order: paramedics (or other emergency rescue)
first, then anything else.

Fire Extinguisher

One of those small, hand ones. No home should be without one,
particularly not yours right now. They are the least exciting way to
deal with fires, and no one at your home needs extra excitement.

Medication

See the entry on page 110.

All measures aim at an immediate atmosphere in your home of confidence, assurance, and, above all, normality to establish in every way that the patient truly is no longer a patient. A doctor, remembering his own days as a patient, stresses the need "to help make the patient feel less dependent and more in control." For the family, that means not mincing about for fear of "upsetting" someone with a heart condition. It means getting back to normal.

Even if normality means, as one nurse puts it, "finding a way to argue, a way to let off steam and frustration," the result is an increase in your ability to give needed support. Dr. Manuel Straker's wife had heart surgery, so he speaks with double authority since his specialty is psychiatry. Recuperating patients need a lot of support, especially from their spouses. But those spouses, Dr. Straker says,

> . . . may not be able to supply that support if they themselves are overwhelmed by resentful feelings toward the sick spouse—who may be a burden, a worry, who may not be able to carry the full weight that the spouse expects them to.
>
> Also, it's emotionally draining to be with, to listen to, someone who's sick and complaining and upset a lot.
>
> Spouses need an opportunity to sound off and unburden—maybe at first to the doctor or nurse—to allow these feelings to surface, to come face-to-face with them. Otherwise they remain buried and denied and they fester.
>
> Then, after the spouse can acknowledge these feelings and express them, it may be very useful to have the two people talk about it together, because the sick person is very well aware of what the spouse is feeling, and if it isn't out in the open, may very well respond with retaliatory anger, or guilt, or all kinds of other destructive emotions.

Normal family relationships should constitute the emotional atmosphere for recovery.

Doing Things

First, when the patient remains homebound *by doctor's orders* you should constantly encourage activities that strongly smack of building for the future. Entertainment or plain distraction have their place, and are easy enough to arrange, what with TV (plus VCRs and movie rentals) and the easy availability of light reading, hobbies, even games and puzzles. But activities that involve learning something new or otherwise improving your patient's future position—those are golden. It is the difference between doing a crossword puzzle and learning to play bridge, between reading a novel and a book that will improve the patient's poker game, between watching a movie on

VCR and watching an instructional tape in the patient's field (or a new, better one!). You get the idea.

As soon as your patient can circulate, the activity you promote is . . . *activity*.

Polly Brown neatly sums it up:

> If they stay in the house all the time, they'll get bored and depressed. They have to get outside—and not just with the spouse. I've had too many patients call me and say, "Well, I just don't feel well; I hurt all over."
>
> I say, "What have you been doing?" It turns out they've been hanging around home, with the spouse. A typical conversation goes like this:
>
> I ask, "Why hasn't your wife gone back to work? Why isn't she saving that time off, so when you feel better in three or four weeks, you can do something together for a week, when you're feeling good?"
>
> "Well, you told her that, but she thinks she has to stay home with me."
>
> "She doesn't have to stay home with you; you're perfectly all right. You're fine. Tell her to get on back to work. Start planning what you're going to do when you feel good. Get away if you can. If you can't, at least do things with friends when you have strength to do it."

Come to think, what better for-the-future activity could there be than *planning* a trip—itinerary, routes, transportation, reservations for accommodations, things to do, sights to see, the works. And if it's to a foreign country, out come the language books and tapes!

Exercise (Also see chapter 13, "Rehabilitation")

The doctor almost surely has prescribed a course of exercise with flexible limits.* Ideally, a rehab program is supervising a formal program. The better doctors and hospitals consciously and progressively banish any patient anxiety over the "safety" of exercise before discharge. "We start exercise the first day in the ICU," says Dr. Allan Lansing. "Simple things with arms and legs. It's a positive approach: 'Yes, I can move my arms and legs; *yes*, I can sit up; *yes*, I can walk.'" And before going home, yes, I can ride a stationary bike—plainly more taxing than any exercise the doctor has prescribed, so what I'm doing *has* to be safe.

The benefits of exercise are enormous, from the obvious ones such as weight control, rebuilding strength, stamina, and "wind," to more

---

* "Twice a day, walk around the block at least twice, and keep going until you get tired, but no more than 10 times until I see you again, and don't lift anything you can't hold easily in one hand." That sort of thing.

subtle ones such as lowering cholesterol and keeping the patient, one doctor says, "from bogging down in introspection." The risk of exercise is minimal; therapists can show even those who are impaired ways to exercise that safely conserve energy. Dr. Frederick Grover clearly specifies the goal of exercise:

> If at all possible, patients ought to get back to normal activity and do the things they think are fun—even if there may be a slight amount of risk—for the psychological good of it. That's why we do the operations: to get people back to normal.
>
> Now, if they have incomplete vascularization, still have angina, obviously they can't; but if they're rendered asymptomatic, as 85 to 95% of them will be, they can get back to their occupations and avocations.

Dr. Hillel Laks states flatly,

> All patients, after bypass surgery, should be on a daily, or five-times-a-week exercise program for a minimum of 20 minutes, preferably an hour a day if that's possible, as a permanent part of their program.

What kind of exercise program should your patient follow? For a choice, one tailored by rehab specialists or the cardiologist. (*Important:* If you have to invent your own program, at least check it with the doctor.) General guidelines exist. Exercise should be aerobic rather than isometric—steady, repetitive motions that require the body to keep burning oxygen, not actions that suddenly strain muscles for a short period, such as weight lifting. Golf three times a week, a rehab expert points out, is not enough—which too many people don't realize. Dr. Harvey Alpern says,

> The proper type of exercise is whatever you enjoy and will do that's aerobic—swimming, jogging, riding a stationary bike, jumping rope, whatever you enjoy.
>
> Tennis would be fine, but a lot of time is spent standing around. You want some activity that's relatively continuous to bring your heart rate up at least 60%, and perhaps 70% of maximal predicted heart rate for about 20 minutes at least four days a week.*
>
> You can do it by walking—progressive walking, farther and faster as time goes on. There are tables and forms that indicate how to do this.

One interesting wrinkle for walking is the use of shopping malls, heated in winter, air conditioned in summer, with "scenery" for the easily bored. Some malls open early specially for groups of heart walkers, with markers to let walkers know how far they've gone on any given circuit.

---

* One of the best, easy-to-understand texts we've seen is "Walking for Fitness," an 8-page pamphlet from Krames Communications. See "Reading Materials," below, for details.

Exercise should be structured as to seem more fun than a chore. "I know for myself," says Polly Brown, "I get home at night and I'm tired, I don't want to 'exercise.' However, if someone says, C'mon, we're going dancing—suddenly I've got all the energy in the world." It helps if exercise becomes integral to family life. Brown also says, "one of may favorite times of the day, still, is late twilight when Daddy and I would just go walking. It was special, a treat; but everybody was doing it, not just my father."

The family that walks together, talks together—and you can take it from there.

Light Bulb Problems

Another piece of nomenclature that we at first thought outdated stems from the weakness and muscle atrophy that regularly attend long hospital stays. The name comes from our own stock of Things We Wish We Had Known.

Two days out of the hospital, JoAnn's husband decided to replace a burned-out light bulb. When he found that his hospital stay had left him too weak even to unscrew the light bulb, he was sick with frustration, and all the more determined to *change that damned bulb*. Another 15 minutes found Forrest even weaker, plus exhausted. Enter JoAnn. She saw her husband sitting with new light bulb in hand (gathering strength for another assault; but how was she to know?), malevolently eyeing a burned-out bulb that, to him, seemed welded in place. Wanting to "help," she sweetly took the bulb out of Forrest's hand and blithely started to make the switch—an operation that came to a sudden end as Forrest exploded.

His rage was nature's way of saying, "Get lost, I need the exercise."

Within whatever physical limits the doctor or therapist has decreed at the start, the harder something is to do, the more important it is for a patient to keep trying. It's like a baby learning to walk, or anyone who has suffered a sudden, crippling handicap relearning lost skills. "Helping" either one, far from a kindness, would constitute the most pitiless sort of meddling in a necessary and natural process, no matter how hard the "struggle" seemed to be.

We knew the principle held good, but we assumed such weakness was a thing of the past (this was in the mid-1960s) along with 6-week hospital stays and severely limited exercise.

Not so. "The doctor said we could go for walks or rides," says Mrs. R, "but Hank didn't have any energy at first." "They showed us a film at the hospital," says Mrs. V, "and I remember it said, You're going to be tired and so forth. But he would say to me, 'Should I be *this* tired?'"

The answer is still, "Yes," especially for those who had been sick a fair while before treatment. "The only thing that stands out in my mind," one transplant patient said,

> is that I was weaker than hell. I thought I was going to be much stronger, but I was so weak that if I lifted my hands above my head to wash my hair, it just exhausted me. And I thought, "Hey I have a new heart; so why can't I just get up and, like, *run*?"

The weakness passes, more quickly today than before. Meanwhile, keep your hands off those light bulbs.

Medication

Even though your home is not a hospital, you should faithfully follow one hospital routine without disguise: keeping a record of medication. Actually, your patient should, eventually, but you'll have to inaugurate and maintain it until your patient is up to the task.

Prepare a chart (see page 111 for a sample) of the exact medication and exact, day-to-day dosage required (hour-by-hour, if the doctor so specifies). Keep it unmovably near the medication supply, with a pen or pencil firmly attached. Make it an inviolable rule to check off each medication as it comes out of its container, especially "every-four-hours-or-after-meals" medicines. Even for transplant patients, one dose missed or one too many may not spell disaster, but is worrisome and entirely unnecessary.

To help, you can buy a plastic pill box with seven separate compartments, each marked with a day of the week. Load the week's budget of medication at one time and you always know two things: when you're running out, and whether all of today's pills were taken.

Also keep separate, in a travel kit, at least a three-day supply of every medication, rotating the supply with each fresh batch bought. Although it's principally for emergencies—to snatch up and take with you in a fire or earthquake—it also helps you avoid the otherwise inevitable Sunday evening scramble to find an open drugstore when you discover that someone miscounted or forgot, and the coumadin or prednisone has run out.

Reading Material

Titles of pamphlets and booklets are in quotes (e.g., "Walking for Fitness"); book titles are in italic type (e.g., *American Heart Association Cookbook*). For those we discuss elsewhere in the book, we give the page number after the reference.

Medication and Dosage	Monday	Tuesday	Wednesday	Thursday	Friday	Saturday	Sunday	Week of
	AM Noon PM	AM Noon PM	AM Noon PM	AM Noon PM	AM Noon PM	AM Noon PM	AM Noon PM	
	AM Noon PM	AM Noon PM	AM Noon PM	AM Noon PM	AM Noon PM	AM Noon PM	AM Noon PM	
	AM Noon PM	AM Noon PM	AM Noon PM	AM Noon PM	AM Noon PM	AM Noon PM	AM Noon PM	
	AM Noon PM	AM Noon PM	AM Noon PM	AM Noon PM	AM Noon PM	AM Noon PM	AM Noon PM	
	AM Noon PM	AM Noon PM	AM Noon PM	AM Noon PM	AM Noon PM	AM Noon PM	AM Noon PM	
	AM Noon PM	AM Noon PM	AM Noon PM	AM Noon PM	AM Noon PM	AM Noon PM	AM Noon PM	
	AM Noon PM	AM Noon PM	AM Noon PM	AM Noon PM	AM Noon PM	AM Noon PM	AM Noon PM	
Weight								

Clinic visit:

Next appointment:

Comments:

Heart Beat: A Complete Guide to Understanding & Preventing Heart Disease (by Emmanuel Horovitz, M.D.; Health Trends Publishing, P.O. Box 17420, Encino CA 91416, 1988) (see page 42)

"Walking for Fitness" (Krames Communications, 312 90th St., Daly City, CA 94015 (415) 994-8800) (see page 108)

"A Guide to Managing Stress" (Krames Communications, address above)

American Heart Association Cookbook (4th Edition; David McKay Publishers, Inc., New York, 1984) (see page 126)

Craig Claiborne's Gourmet Diet (by Craig Claiborne with Pierre Franey; Times Books, New York, 1980) (see page 126)

Harriet Roth's Cholesterol Control Cookbook (New American Library, New York, 1989) (see page 126)

Seafood: A Collection of Heart-Healthy Recipes (by Janis Harsila, R.D., and Evie Hansen; National Sea Food Educators, P.O. Box 60006, Richmond Beach, WA 98160) (see page 126)

Cooking à la Heart (Mankato Heart Health Program, 101 N. 2nd St., Suite 202, Mankato, MN 56001) (see page 127)

The American Way of Life Need Not Be Hazardous to Your Health (by John Farquhar; Addison-Wesley, 1987)

Charts and Booklets on Food Additives and Nutrition (Center for Science and Public Interest, 1501 16th Street, N.W., Washington, DC 20036) (see page 132)

The following pamphlets are available from the American Heart Association. Consult your local chapter.

"The American Heart Association Diet": An Eating Plan for Healthy Americans (see page 127)

"Cholesterol and Your Heart" (see page 127)

"Dining Out": A Guide to Restaurant Dining (see page 127)

"Heart Facts" (Note: We used "1988 Heart Facts"; the 1989 edition is now available, and there will be periodic updates)

"Heart Attack and Stroke": Signals and Action

"Aspirin and Your Heart"

"Dine to Your Heart's Content": Restaurant Program (see page 137; listing of restaurants serving "coronary cuisine" in your area; this differs from "Dining Out," above, which is general information about eating in any restaurant)

"Nutritious Nibbles": A Guide to Healthy Snacking (see page 135)

"Nutrition for the Fitness Challenge" (see page 135)

"Nutrition Labeling" Food Selection Hints for Fat-Controlled Meals (see page 135)

"Recipes for Low-Fat, Low-Cholesterol Meals" (see page 135; a selection from The *American Heart Association Cookbook*)

In addition, check your chapter of the American Heart Association for their list of other available reading materials.

Social Life, Your

For most, the hospital stay is now too short for "getting away" to become so overwhelmingly necessary. However, that period combined with the length of time before the patient gets out of the house may raise the problem.

"It's important for the family, particularly the spouse, to try to maintain some sense of normal life," says Ruth Lusk, a transplant group coordinator, "rather than staying there, concentrating on the patient 24 hours a day, 7 days a week." It doesn't matter what you do, she says,

> . . . go shopping, get your hair done, go play golf—just get away for a couple of hours to get your objectivity back. It's important for the spouse, the family, a brother or sister, children, whoever it is, because you can't help the patient the way you should if you get tired and lose your objectivity.

Don't worry that the patient will resent your absence. Your regaining of objectivity, of a breathing spell, is a positive aid. As a member of Lusk's group put it,

> You forget what's normal if you don't get away. And I think it flows over to the patient. If I can come back in from 18 holes of golf and tell Jack my score—and all the "but I should have hads, I could have hads, if I'd onlys"—why, he laughs and smiles. You're bringing back something from the outside.

The main thing you bring back is a more balanced you.

Visitors

All-in-all, visitors are welcome as the flowers of spring, even counting the occasional thorn. They approximate natural contacts with the normal world, another step toward adjustment and total recovery. Indeed, the wife of one patient counts it a prime responsibility of the family to "find people who will interact well with the patient and keep everyone's spirits up."

Overdoing constitutes the only problem: seeing too many people too soon, staying up too late, getting tired—not even in a constructive physical way, as with exercise. Trouble is, the patient may not feel tired and visitors may not perceive the tiredness. Everyone is having such a good time!

It's up to you to control matters, something best done ahead of time so as to avoid scenes. Mrs. C's husband was 75 years old, popular, with lots of friends both social and professional. She made a flat rule that only one couple could visit a night, and enforced it for the six weeks of home recuperation. Almost all the friends understood, as what true friends would not?

You can also impose some time limits beforehand, telling the visitors how long they should stay. When the time's up, most will go. You can privately make it known to oafs who overstay their time that they won't be welcome if it happens again.

A word on serving refreshments. Consensus is against any elaboration; but that obviously depends on how you and the patient feel about it. Tea, coffee, cookies, wine, a drink; that's probably no big deal for anyone involved, and it contributes to the proper festivity of the visit. Much beyond that is probably unwise (absent a *strong* feeling on the part of the patient about wanting to seem a more gracious host or hostess); it will simply encourage longer, possibly wearing, stays; what's more, most party food tends not to be part of a sound coronary diet, making it hard for the patient either way.

If you remember the distinction between these visits and purely social occasions you cannot go far wrong. These are a form of therapy, part of the recovery process. The more light-hearted aspects of having friends in must not interfere with rest or diet, or your relationship with the patient.

Weaning Anxiety, More

A number of important differences, good and bad, distinguish this from the variety some patients experience in the hospital when moved from a CCU or ICU to a regular floor.

On the bad side, any apprehension about the move home contains more substance. Help is not down the hall; it's a phone call and ambulance ride away.

Nevertheless, any patient has to be glad to get out of a hospital. Furthermore, the visible difference between the high-tech special care unit and a regular hospital room is much greater than the difference between that room and home.

What can aggravate any tendency toward weaning anxiety now is expressed or perceived anxiety on *your* part. As nurse-coordinator Kim Wimsatt puts it,

> I want the family to realize that when they go home not to walk on egg shells, and not to worry at every twinge, that they have to rush the patient to the emergency room. I want them to feel confident and comfortable with this situation.

Education does it. If you're lucky, that's already taken care of in the hospital. Patient and family have received complete, persuasive briefings on the patient's condition and what it means. Wimsatt continues:

> When you tell them what they can or can't do when they go home, they say, "I can *really* do that? I can really take a walk? We can really go on this trip? We can go out on the lake?" They want almost a list of, "Yes, I can walk; I can eat this, I can't eat that; I can lift this, I can't lift that."
>
> If the family doesn't get this information, they're really anxious about taking the patient home. They're more secure with the patient still being in the hospital because they don't know what to do; if something went wrong, they wouldn't know how to handle it.
>
> If you go in there and tell them what to expect, they're eager to go home, and they're ready to handle the situation.

If the professionals at your hospital did not volunteer such information, insist on getting it with your patient, preferably before going home, certainly as soon as possible. And have a paper and pen ready to take notes. That should reduce anxiety on everyone's part.

Whole Family Involved

The whole family must play a part for best possible recovery. It's more than the immediately obvious. Walking (or otherwise exercising) together and eating the same food are important; a consciousness that, "We're all part of this"—and what flows from that realization—are even more important.

As the daughter of one patient says, "The relationship changes a little; the child becomes more like a parent; I felt it was my turn to give *him* support and encouragement now." And to give a sort of parental intervention. Her father tended toward gruffness, was impatient with his own now-necessary dependence. The woman was "afraid he'd take it out on Mom." She took it on herself to talk about it with her father: "It's hard on you," she said, "but it's hard on Mom, too." He should keep that in mind. As, in fact, he did.

In another family, the key to bucking up the morale of a woman facing catheterization was a visit from an uncle who drove many miles to say he'd had one, himself, and to assure her that it wasn't so bad. The patient's mother, who sensed what it would mean to have reassurance from *family* (despite the deluge of reassurance by the professionals) arranged the uncle's trip.

In both examples, these were adults, but the help and enlistment of the family has nothing to do with age. All can play a part, and one of the greatest parts you can play is to recruit and coordinate their help. Then *none* of you is alone.

CHAPTER 9

Personality Change

Complaint, Nature of the

I know from *Survive** that it's almost traditional for heart patients to go through certain problems like this. Joe was a classic case. He had all of them.

You know him; you know him to be a very nice person. He became an absolute monster after that operation. He just turned into a completely self-indulgent, angry, demanding person. It continued for months after surgery; in fact it got worse and worse. He became more self-involved.

It was a personality change—to such an extent, that we broke up for a couple of years.

—Mrs. O

I get a lot of concerned phone calls from families wanting some explanation of why he's so irritable—the slightest little thing sets him off, whereas he used to be such an easygoing guy.

They can't understand what could have caused that kind of behavioral change. They can't believe it's a normal process.

—Dr. John Strobeck

It takes many forms, though hostility and "touchiness" are the most common. It can be sexual, as in The Grand Turk Syndrome we

---

* Mr. and Mrs. O are friends of ours. Mr. O had a bypass operation in 1981. Doctors diagnosed his condition before he had a heart attack. Mrs. O read our first book, *Survive*, during the period of the problems she describes.

116

mentioned. Whatever the specifics of aberrant behavior, the one constant is the family's observation that "this isn't *like*" the person they know.

In the era of weeks-long hospital stays, any personality change used to surface toward the end of the hospital stay, when patients had gotten over the shock of discovery, fear of immediate death, and gratitude that it hadn't happened. They then had time to ponder their situation. And—wham! One wife, back then, complained:

> My husband changed. His personality changed, and he was wild! . . .
> He was ordering everybody around and complaining all the time he was in the hospital. I kept saying, "This isn't like him."
> . . . He'd have me move everything around in the room and I had to fix the bed just so. Once, three women he works with came to visit, and he had them change the room all around again.
> . . . Twice I went away crying because he'd been so mean. "Fix my bed this way—NOT that way. THIS way!"
> He had never talked to me like that!

Now the onset more likely occurs at home. The result remains the same.

Patients aren't usually aware of a behavior change in themselves, but evidence suggests that they are aware of the underlying cause. The husband of Mrs. O, the woman quoted at the beginning of this chapter, says,

> There's a great rage: people don't know this except those who've had heart operations or heart attacks. You have a rage for several months, great anger. I thought I was going out of my head, I got so angry.
> Maybe the mind knows that the body has been violated. But you get furious at very little things.

Neither rage nor reaction is restricted to male patients. Mr. F says,

> It was tough at first. She'd be saying, "You're sweet putting up with me"—then turn around and just pow! for nothing: because you dropped a crumb on the floor.
> You say, "Hey! back off, ease up."
> Then they *really* light into you: you're accusing them of being unreasonable, which they are being, but they can't see it.
> Then maybe a half hour later they say, "I don't know what happened to me."

Enemy, You are the (Who, me?)

> I concentrated on telling myself this wasn't my fault, that this wasn't him, that all this hostility was not *really* directed at me. I worked very hard at not taking it personally.

But I did take it personally after a while. I thought he hated me. I became convinced that he wanted me out of his life. He seemed to resent my wanting to help. The more I tried, the more he pushed away. I truly thought he hated me. So that was the end. I left.

—Mrs. O

With hostility, as with shopping, the rule remains: Don't go to strangers when you can deal with those you know.

True, patients might more properly direct the rage they feel against Fate or chance or heredity or saturated fats or conniving business associates—whatever they decide brought on the heart condition. But those do not make very satisfactory targets. No one can rage against Fate (or even cholesterol) for very long; you soon crave a more pliable, more vulnerable, more responsive target. That, classically, is how cats get kicked. Also families.

What's more, you and the family are at hand. You are familiar; it's easier to pick quarrels and to hurt those you know.

Spouses are usually the favored target. ("I remember," says Mrs. O, "another woman saying her father had gone through it. He almost literally threw his wife out the door, and they had been married 40 years or something.") But no one in the family is immune. Mr. O had children from a previous marriage; one daughter lived in the same city. "Louise really suffered," Mrs. O says. "Joe was terribly abusive with her; not as much as with me, but poor Louise really suffered during that period."

Prevalence and Duration

I used to talk with other women who had gone through similar ordeals, and they all agreed: it's a phenomenon that occurs. That was proof to me that it's common to all heart patients.

—Mrs. O

Not all, by any means. Nor does the personality change strike with equal severity all those who suffer it. If it doesn't happen, or only very mildly, with the person you love, count yourself lucky; if it does . . . well, now you know what's happening.

How long will it last? Aside from Mr. O (who, as you'll see in "Reasons," below, suffered a crushing and extraordinary collection of reasons to feed ongoing rage), the longest period of personality change we've heard of lasted only a couple of months. That was part of Mrs. O's distraction over the situation. From *Survive* and other women she talked with, she kept thinking it would be over any day. When, as she says, "it went on for months and months and months," she lost hope, and finally separated from her husband in despair of his ever again being himself. We look at the outcome in "What To Do," below.

Reasons for It

I don't know why. Do you?

—Mrs. O

No one can know for sure, but we can make persuasive guesses.

Surely a large part derives from the sudden, scarring intimation of mortality we examined in chapter 7 ("Psychological Reaction"), plus the shock of realization that one's lifestyle must surely change in some ways (and the uncertainty of what ways they may be), the fear that one may not be able to care for the family as well (or at all), that the illness may cripple one's career—leading inevitably to guilt over having, by omission or commission, brought all this upon oneself and one's family.

Add the universal cry of "Why *me*?," that howl against manifest injustice, and the wonder is not that many heart patients suffer a temporary personality change, but that they don't all run amok.

"I used to think, How can Joe survive all this?" says Mrs. O,

He's had bypass surgery, he's been diagnosed with diabetes, he's realized he has a drinking problem so he's given that up and joined AA, his partner has done bad things to him so his business has gone to pieces, his wife has left him, he's had to quit smoking. And then he found out that his medical insurance was no good.

Is it surprising that Mr. O's anger lasted somewhat longer than most?

We saw in "Enemy," above, the reason that patients direct hostility most vividly toward spouses and the rest of the family. But another reason more closely approaches the center of the problem. No emotionally mature adult likes dependence, yet patients suddenly find themselves in the most dependent of roles: being weak, sick, and needing. The position particularly galls men—who, as one nurse observes on page 97, will often, when they start feeling better, "pick a quarrel just in order to take the upper hand again." A doctor notes the same phenomenon with both men and women. For the first few post-hospital visits, the spouse accompanies the patient (often because the patient needs help); then the dual visits usually stop. "Patients," he says, "no longer want company; it's protecting an image of themselves as independent."

Seen in that light, hostility, even when directed at you, is a healthy sign of recovery, evidence that your patient is struggling to get back to normal. Too bad it can't be a pleasanter sign.

What To Do About It

> I guess I would have to say what my friend said and what your book said: Be patient; stick it out; he doesn't hate you; he doesn't mean what he's saying. I wish I had understood it better at the time; I might have been wiser about it.
>
> —Mrs. O

Because Mr. O's hostility and personality change lasted such a long time, reading in *Survive* that it constituted an almost expected phenomenon didn't help any more than a friend's similar assurance could. Mrs. O felt sure that *this* was different; *this* was permanent. But Mrs. O's experience serves as an important gloss on what you read here: even if your case is somehow unusual, the basic principle remains the same. This, too, even *this*, shall pass.

Assuming that, unlike Mrs. O, you do not despair and separate (if a spouse) or leave home (if another family member), you meanwhile have a choice of three things to do.

RETALIATE: Fight back, give as good as you get.

IGNORE IT: Close your ears to nastiness, your eyes and feelings to meanness.

MAKE FLEXIBLE ADJUSTMENT: Within the limits of human nature be as forbearing as possible and as reasonable as possible in loving correction.

Retaliation is satisfying. It's only human to hit back at someone who hit first—and unjustly, at that! While his wife was recovering, Mr. F cultivated the art of, as he says, "letting it go by" as much as possible. But, he says,

> This is difficult to keep doing; sometimes I'd have a bad day, then— whooo! I would lash back occasionally. "Why do I have to put up with you all the time and you don't have to put up with me?"

Was the lashing back beneficial? Was it good for Mrs. F to get back some of what she was inflicting? "I don't know," says Mr. F with a laugh, "but it was sure good for me; I felt great." They share a warm, strong, long-enduring marriage; besides, the backlash came only on occasion. More fragile relationships could shatter, especially if thrust and counterthrust become routine. Moreover, steady retaliation can only put bounce and vigor into a conflict that might otherwise peter out.

Perpetually just "taking it," on the other hand, can almost as readily sour a relationship. It breeds a sense of martyrdom that you may later find hard to forgive. Anyway, how can you keep a bland smile while your teeth are clenched?

The best course is a balance. Years ago, one wife gave us a workable formula:

> I have to be better-natured, more understanding of the times when he reacts. But no matter what I tell myself, I'm still human, and there are still going to be . . . *times!*

Good nature, patience, love, perception, understanding. And the greatest of these is all of them, with maybe a slight edge for understanding—not just of why the patient turns hostile and into a different person, but also of yourself, a human being. The same wife went on to say,

> There are times when I feel that he's "flexing his muscles" a little bit, and I hope to be in a mood to be sensitive, to be wise enough to know this is simply that kind of expression. I don't always know. Sometimes I react, and I don't always remember that he's sick.
>
> I'm very sensitive. And when somebody's harsh with me, I don't like it. And if he's harsh with me out of his own needs, and I forget momentarily what's causing it—you know, it's like any relationship: I may snap back. We may have words.

So what? All members of every family "have words" from time to time, heart condition or no. It's another aspect of normal life to which the entire family must reaccustom itself. The trick is to mix forbearance and firm refusal to be trampled. When the patient becomes outrageous, if you understand yourself and your emotional needs, you can lovingly say just that. He or she is being unreasonable and hurting you; you are not happy about it and will not quietly stand for it.

Two affirmative acts will also help:

GET OUT: Give the patient some time alone, time to miss you, time to talk sense to himself (it's received better from that source, anyway).

GET OTHERS IN: Other faces help the process of normalizing behavior and generally force a restoration of civility: it's harder to be impossible with friends in for a visit. As one wife puts it, "when they were there, my husband was fine! [LAUGHING] He only complained, and was miserable, around us!"

Mr. O's case was extreme, and Mrs. O's "getting out" was equally so: a separation that started about a year after the surgery, when his personality change and hostility continued. Did it help? "Definitely!" says Mrs. O,

> I'm not patting myself on the back, because I didn't do it for that reason, but I think it was therapeutic. It was absolutely essential that Joe be left alone at that time. He needed to crawl into a shell and be left alone by the whole world, having nothing to worry about, nothing

to think about. He could not cope with—well, feeding the animals! It was more than he could do.

He needed a period of peace without any responsibility, not even the responsibility of having someone around who took care of him—and cared for him. I'm sure he must have been conscious of the fact that he was being a monster. So it would have helped him to have that guilt removed. I would have represented the guilt to him, I'm sure.

What happened while he was in retreat from the world? "He did an awful lot of soul-searching," says Mrs. O.

He took an honest look at himself—and as he had become and as he had been. And he said, "I don't like what I see, and I'm going to change."

It was hard for him to do because he had always had a volatile personality. He just kept it under wraps. He was always at the point of exploding, and frequently did. He just willed himself to get rid of that; it doesn't exist anymore.

We had been separated, and for a year hadn't seen each other. Then we slowly started seeing each other again, and I began to be aware that he was a different person altogether. He was different, even, from what he had been prior to the change. He had become very, very introspective and gentle. He had absolutely willed himself to stop being a high-pressure person.

He's a completely different person now.

They got back together, moved to a smaller, less hectic, less expensive community, making it easier for Mr. O to renounce his high-pressure profession. Today they live contented and happy. Mr. O takes his insulin for diabetes, neither smokes nor drinks, keeps his weight down, and has experienced no recurrence of heart problems.

Mrs. O realizes that separation is not the answer or at all necessary for most couples. In the more extreme cases, while the personality change rages, she advises with a mischievous smile,

If you have the money, maybe take a cruise around the world. Separately.

Actually, the occasional trip around the block should do it nicely for you and the rest of the family.

CHAPTER 10

Food—for Eating and Thought

All Together	Fat	Out, Eating
Attitude	Labels, Reading	Own Program,
Cookbooks	Learn, What to	Creating Your
Cooking	and Where to	Salt/Sodium
Fads	Moderation	Summing Up

Patients can't do it on their own. They can't eat the way they must if all the other food put on the table is the wrong kind. The whole family has to understand that everybody in the family will benefit from eating the right way. And they all have to be participants.

—Dr. Allan Lansing

All Together

Why should it be an issue? A wife tells us, "I can't follow Don around to see what he eats. But he knows that if he eats wrong and something happens, it hurts me, too. He knows how important he is to me, and I'm important to him, so we do this together." One patient calls it, "a partnership in being sensible." Surely everyone in the family deserves healthy food. A doctor declares, "*certainly* the children of a patient who has had coronary artery disease should be eating the kinds of food we know can reduce cholesterol levels." Another doctor, when trying to convince families that they must all change their eating habits, cites those Korean War autopsy studies (see chapter 3), showing the shocking prevalence of clogged arteries in American young people.

Small wonder adolescent arteries clog. A 1988 Gallup poll revealed that while 94% of our teenagers "know they should eat a low cholesterol diet," and almost half would like to, they don't know good foods from bad. Almost a third don't know that eggs have anything to do with cholesterol; over two-thirds don't know that ice cream is involved. Few schools teach nutrition; worse, their lunchrooms actively promote raging cholesterol levels because foods whose calories come from high fat and high sugar are easy to prepare, popular, and inexpensive. "To save money," says a doctor, "they are serving this type of food to the kids. It's a national disgrace!"

The dangers of heredity apply to "children" of every age. When the wife of a bypass patient decided to eat the same way as her husband now did, she says her own doctor was delighted because she had lost both parents to heart disease.

When the whole family eats "right," results gratify. Beyond making compliance infinitely easier for the patient, the whole family's weight problems often disappear. "With one fellow," says rehab nurse, Pam Moore,

> his daughter lost 30 pounds in four or five months. The wife felt a little low because she wasn't losing as fast as everybody else. They walk every morning, developing closeness in the family, a willingness to share. A lot of times the people this happens to—it's difficult for them to share their feelings. This can bring them together, to share, and to learn that it's OK to have feelings.

Another nurse, Kevan Shaheen, says, "I know families who think it's *odd* that people eat 'fast food,' and make the wrong choices when they do: they're so used to eating the right way at home."

The patient, incidentally, must participate in this concept of "all together." That may seem a strange point to make, since it starts with the patient; but if that patient is a man, particularly one who came to maturity before, say, 1960, it can be a problem. Mention nutrition to a male patient of 55 or so, and all to often you hear, "Well, talk to the cook, over there." Humana enforces a firm rule: "We have wives," says Kevan Shaheen,

> who come in and want to get instructions for their husbands—and we *don't* allow that. We encourage the cooking-shopping person to come in, too. But it's an individual choice issue, and responsibility. We encourage each of the family members to take responsibility for their own health.

Sue Rogers, clinical dietitian at Humana, tells male patients, "She doesn't feed you every bite you eat, so you need to know what choices to make when she's not around." "That," Rogers says,

> puts the responsibility onto the person himself. It also helps ease some feelings of over-responsibility for the wife. I have some who said, "Last week I fed him such-and-such; did that cause this? I've been feeding him since he left his mother's house; did I do this to him?" They're *so* guilt-laden.

Usually I'll say something along the lines of, "Diet is not the only risk factor; and, anyway, you didn't cook every meal that he ate."

A lot of time the wives feel, "It's *my* responsibility to prevent this from happening again" with the way they cook. I think that's out of perspective: they can be conscientious and supportive, but to assume that they, alone, can prevent what's wrong with their husband isn't fair. So turning to patients and putting some responsibility on them should free the wife to say, "Yeah! wait a minute: it's his body, his life, his mouth, so it's his choice; I can do supportive things. But I'm not solely responsible."

She notes a distinctly greater willingness among younger men to share that responsibility.

It's up to you to make sure that your patient, as well as every family member of every age and both genders, all start to share responsibility for his or her own health, and the communal family health!

Attitude

Except when quoting others, we conscientiously avoid the word "diet." Anyone who has ever been on a diet knows what it means: deprivation, hunger (especially for forbidden foods), willpower (or guilt), fussy, finicky meal preparation, temptation. A diet is something you must constantly "watch." A diet is hell. And that's when it lasts only a month or so. How about a lifetime?

The concept of "diet" suggests a goal: we'll abide our deprivations until the scale reads a certain figure—then (too often) whoopee! What your patient and you and the entire family need has as its "goal" no number or even quantifiable result; you seek, rather, a healthy, constructive way of eating for the rest of your lives. We're not talking diet but lifestyle.

Nothing about it mandates deprivation, unappetizing food, or tasteless food preparation, not even for the sterner requirements of diabetics. Eating right simply becomes your family's habit. One struggles with a diet; eating habits come easy, the reflection of natural inclination. In a remarkably short while the family eats right because that's what they're used to. As one woman told us about her children, "Now that they're young adults, they don't think of it as self-discipline even. It's natural to them now."

Only this attitude makes the right kind of family eating possible, not to mention easy and satisfying.

Cookbooks

There are now so many good cookbooks with gourmet recipes that are low-cholesterol, low-fat, and low-sodium for cardiac patients that it's easy to cook for good health for everybody, including your children.

—Dr. Frederick Grover

Once again, the bible is:

The American Heart Association Cookbook (4th ed., David McKay Publishers, Inc., NY, 1984).

They were unaccountably slow in coming out with a low-sodium version, but this edition is it—authoritative, comprehensive, with guidance for shopping, cooking, and serving meals, plus of course a wealth of recipes. Available most book stores.

For cooking artistry, and a positive treasure for everyone on a specifically low-sodium diet is:

Craig Claiborne's Gourmet Diet (Craig Claiborne with Pierre Franey, Times Books, New York, 1980)

Easily America's premier restaurant critic, long for *The New York Times,* Claiborne trained as a chef and brings his *truly* gourmet touch to marvelous recipes. Franey is a chef, and currently writes for the *Times.* The recipes are so good that if you had to choose between cooking with Claiborne and with salt, goodbye salt. Available most book stores (also in paperback).

Right in line with current concerns about cholesterol, the definitive book is:

Harriet Roth's Cholesterol Control Cookbook (New American Library, New York, 1989)

Here you will be treated to the "user friendliest" course in creative, healthy, yet sumptuous cooking by the former Director of the Pritikin Longevity Center Cooking School. Her presentation confirms that the healthy route need not be tedious, tasteless, or boring. Chock full of important dietary information, hearty, recipes and special menus. Available most bookstores.

Specifically for fish, by the wives of two fishermen:

Seafood: A Collection of Heart-Healthy Recipes (Janis Harsila, R.D., and Evie Hansen, National Seafood Educators)

Actually, more than just recipes; tips on buying most kinds of fish and shellfish (e.g., frozen is fine if *fresh:* look for the words "frozen at sea" on the label) and preparing them for cooking. About 150 recipes—easy, quick (20 minutes or less, total, to preparation). Write: National Seafood Educators, P.O. Box 60006, Richmond Beach, WA 98160. $13.95, including postage.

Excellent, 435-recipe book, with menus:

Cooking à la Heart (Mankato Heart Health Program)

Complete nutrition analysis, per portion, for every recipe. Write: Mankato Heart Health Program Foundation, 101 N. Second St., Suite 202, Mankato, MN 56001. $16.70, including postage.

Cooking

No one has to learn anything new or strange to practice what we call "coronary cuisine," whose goal combines maximum reduction of calories, fat, cholesterol, and (usually) sodium, with minimum (often no) reduction in tastiness and dining satisfaction. Proper technique simply means selecting the right skills, maybe adding a few twists of your own. As one wife told us in 1973,

> . . . I have a lot of fun cooking this way—disguising things, changing things, fooling them all! . . . And it really isn't difficult, you know. You take your scissors and take the skin off the chicken and the fat off the meat; you learn to make gravies and skim the fat. . . .
>   Really, I've had a ball!

Many sources offer specific tips and suggestions: the cookbooks listed above contain many; The American Heart Association hands out a number of pamphlets on the subject. Some samples: "The American Heart Association Diet: An Eating Plan for Healthy Americans," "Cholesterol and Your Heart," "Dining Out: A Guide to Restaurant Dining." These and many more are available through your local AHA chapter.

Help positively surrounds even the moderately alert. As we write this, today's food section of a local newspaper points out that if you use chicken in recipes that include some sort of sauce, you can eliminate the skin, which contains the majority of fat, and therefore calories (see "Fat," below), without any discernible diminution of flavor. The article cites, as example, chicken cacciatore*: if the family insists on the chicken's being browned, you can achieve that by lightly brushing the skinned chicken with a bit of olive oil, then broiling, rather than sautéing in the usual three or four tablespoons of oil; otherwise you steam the chicken before adding the other ingredients,

---

* Other skinless delights the article cites: chicken Veronique, paprikash, Marengo, curry, poached with lemons and oranges, grilled with mustard. We are not exactly talking taste deprivation, here, or menu ennui. Fact is, you'll find *roast* skinless chicken entirely palatable, though admittedly different.

further reducing calories and fat. Either way, few palates can detect a difference; after all, the chicken has simmered nearly an hour in flavorsome vegetables, herbs, and spices.

You choose from a hierarchy of alternatives. Often as possible you prepare fish or chicken rather than meat. If meat, you select lean rather than fat-marbled cuts, marinating and broiling with a rack or grilling rather than frying or serving with a sauce. If you must sauté, you use only enough oil to prevent sticking; or use non-stick pans. You always broil or roast with a rack, basting with wine or fruit juice or bouillon rather than drippings. You make stews and gravies enough ahead of time to let the fat form on top, then you skim it off. You substitute yoghurt for all or some sour cream, use skimmed or nonfat milk in "cream" recipes. You use herbs, lemon, and vinegar to enhance vegetables rather than salt, butter, margarine. You cook them in vegetable oil or chicken or beef stock rather than with fatty meats. Where you must use fat, you always choose polyunsaturated oils.

It is fun and the result is tasty.

Fads

Sue Rogers, clinical dietitian, on two of the latest fads, fish oil and oat bran:

> I tend to be conservative on fish oil. I'd like to see a little more research, larger studies done over a longer period of time before I strongly recommend anything for patients. Based on their history, I might say, "If you could eat fish more frequently it may be some help; do it and we'll see what happens." I definitely disagree with fish oil *pills*.
>
> Oat bran looks promising, although studies show you have to eat a lot of it—the equivalent of a bowl of cereal and five muffins a day— to achieve a significant reduction in cholesterol level. And you get the same results from the same quantity of plain oats or dried beans. Studies show that there may be bad side effects from so much. The answer is, as always, you have to check with *your* doctor or nutritionist about *your* needs.

When the medical establishment refuses to mount some hobby horse, the reason is not, as that horse's more fervent backers often suggest, that the establishment reflexively resists progress, squirms with jealousy, or seeks to protect some vested interest. They simply speak with the native caution of professionals who demand a professional level of *proof* before unbridling their enthusiasms.

Not that they necessarily see danger in the substances of the fad; what worries them is the likely substitution of fad for tested treatment. It isn't that cancer doctors worry about patients swallowing ground apricot pits; it's that someone on Laetrile may well abandon, for something unproven, radiation or chemotherapy that's known to be efficacious. "I don't," says Rogers,

> think there's going to be a miracle food that will cure cholesterol problems. Sometimes I see pop or fad diets in the newspapers, and the authors make it sound like, "If you'll just do *this* you'll be OK"—and they haven't mentioned fats at all.

That's the trouble with fads.

When some particular "miracle" proves itself through the sort of rigorous clinical testing that impresses professionals such as Rogers, she and her colleagues will joyously recommend it. Until then, is your family's health and well-being *really* a fit subject for freelance experimentation?

Fat

Start with definitions of the different kinds of fat:

Saturated: Any kind of fat, from any source, that can increase the amount of cholesterol in the bloodstream when eaten in any form.

Cholesterol: A particular kind of saturated fat, found only in animal tissue (and products such as eggs, milk, butter, and cheese). It can raise the cholesterol level in the bloodstream when eaten. (See "Cholesterol," chapter 3).

Monosaturated: A fat that lowers the amount of cholesterol in the bloodstream very slightly.

Polyunsaturated: A fat that lowers the amount of cholesterol in the bloodstream; found only in vegetable matter.

We usually talk about cholesterol measured in milligrams, other fats measured in grams; 1,000 milligrams make a gram, just over 30 grams equal an ounce.

This is vital: one gram of fat contains about 9.3 calories. Compare that with 4 calories per gram of carbohydrate, and you understand why sound weight-loss diets have you fill up on carbohydrates rather than fats. You also understand the on-again-off-again love affair between coronary dietitians and shellfish. Shrimp, crab, and lobster (also scallops, clams, and oysters) contain almost no fat. But what they do have is nearly all cholesterol. For instance,

	Beef	*Shrimp*
Total fat per ounce	5–7 grams	less than ½ gram
Cholesterol per ounce	21 milligrams	38 milligrams

So over the years shellfish swam in and out of official favor, depending on what kind of balance nutritionists currently promoted between cholesterol and total fat intake.

The heart of today's best coronary cuisine theory is the same concept of hierarchical choices that we examined above in "Cooking." You want to reduce fat intake, both in cooking and in selection of foods. Where fat is unavoidable, you choose the polyunsaturates rather than the monosaturates, the monosaturates rather than the saturates. (A new theory suggests that monosaturated fat lowers only LDL, not HDL, so may be preferable to polyunsaturated fat, which lowers both. Check with your nutritionist.) You pick low-fat milk over whole milk, skimmed or nonfat over low-fat. Fortunately, any food label that mentions fat content or cholesterol must give a complete analysis of how much of each kind is in that particular food. If you know the most common sources for each kind of fat, and you

Common Sources of Fat

Kinds of Foods	Kinds of fat they contain			
	Saturated	Cholesterol	Monosat.	Polyunsat.[‡]
Meats	X	X		
Shellfish		X		
Fish	X*			
Poultry	X*			
Eggs		X		
Dairy products	X	X		
Oils[†]				
coconut	X			
cocoa butter	X			
palm	X			
olive			X	
peanut			X	
corn				X
cottonseed				X
safflower				X
sesame seed				X
soybean				X
sunflower seed				X

* Much of the total fat comes away with the skin.
[†] You find them mostly in the form of margarines, cooking oils, and shortenings, and as ingredients in packaged foods.
[‡] If a polyunsaturated oil has been treated to keep it fresh longer it may become a saturated oil. The tip-off words to look for are: hydrogenated, hardened, partially hardened or hydrogenated, stabilized, and specially processed.

recognize the sneakier ways manufacturers try to confuse you (see "Labels, Reading," below) you can make sensible choices. The sources with a significant amount of fat per ounce, plus a couple of important notes, are listed in the table on the opposite page.

In examining your hierarchy of choices, remember two things: the object is to reduce total fat intake; and when it comes to calories, fat is fat, your arteries preferring a gram of corn oil to a gram of palm oil, but your waistline expanding equally with both. "People say, 'Well I only eat chicken,'" says a doctor who, unlike many, keeps abreast of nutrition. "An ounce of chicken has about 77 milligrams of cholesterol, an ounce of lean red meat has maybe 80. So it's not surprising that when people eat huge amounts of chicken they still have problems." Notice, though, that's *lean* red meat.

The deluded say, "Hamburger plainly is not lean, so instead of my usual Big Mac, I'll have the fish sandwich." Don't bother. It's deep fried in fat, and by the time you slather on tartar sauce, you're better off with the hamburger. Or they insist on the *grilled* chicken sandwich—hold the mayo—which they accompany with inevitably greasy French fries. Or, being very good, they go instead to the salad bar, avoiding obvious traps like mayonnaise-larded macaroni and deep-fried croutons, ending with a chaste plate of greens, beans, and vegetables (unmarinated in all that oil). Fine. But what do they douse on it? *Consumer Reports* claims the little pack of Thousand Island dressing McDonald's serves with their salad gives it the calories, due to fat, of a Big Mac. Fat is fat.

None of this means you have to do without. You want a hamburger? Mr. M occasionally buys lean round steak, trims all visible fat, and grinds it up. "Once you get used to a non-juicy hamburger," he says, "it's very tasty." In fact, by now he finds the notion of a *juicy* hamburger—that's the fat running out—repellent. Or content yourself with a small, plain, store-bought burger, insist they leave off the sauce (catsup and mustard are fine), and pile on all the lettuce, tomato, and onion (*not* fried) you want—for a saving of about 150 calories. You know the realities, then choose carefully.

Labels, Reading

We constantly read labels. If Ben has to go to the store, the first thing he does is read labels before he buys something. I have programmed him; I've had to push him into it because it was easier to let me do it. But I said, "We both have to do it." Now he's so label conscious! Sometimes we sound fanatical trying to change our friends.

—Mrs. H

The most sensible approach we've heard on the subject comes from dietitian Mary Bowlby. When asked what questions patients and families ask most, she says,

> They are baffled mostly by labels, so I try to teach logic. If you understand the logic of reading labels, it doesn't matter what product comes out on the market, you should be able to work your way through it.

Here is the logic.

Since 1938, manufacturers have been required to list all the ingredients in processed foods in order of quantity. Since 1975, if the manufacturer mentions fat or cholesterol content (with words like "low fat," "no cholesterol"), or indeed makes any sort of health claim (e.g., "low calorie," "high in polyunsaturates"), the label must include a complete analysis, charts that list size of serving, number of servings in that package, then the calories, cholesterol, fat, sodium, vitamins, etc. per serving.* They tend to use tiny type for listings, so a pocket-sized magnifying glass comes in handy on shopping tours. You may also run across some obscure ingredients; a reference book may be useful. The Center for Science and Public Interest has prepared some fascinating charts and booklets on food additives and nutrition. They are priced at $3.95 each and it just takes a phone call or letter to order: Center for Science and Public Interest, Michael Jacobson, Director, 1501 16th Street N.W., Washington, D.C. 20036 (202) 332-9110.

The logic of checking labels for fat is relatively easy. Even if the label does not account for the number of grams, you can tell if a product contains an unacceptable amount of saturated fat. The rule: the first oil listed must be specified as "liquid." After that, some partially hardened oil probably won't make much difference. If the first oil listed is anything but liquid (or if it's coconut or palm oil or cocoa butter in any form), do not buy that product. This rule makes assessment of any margarine, shortening, cooking oil, and dressing easy. A Heart Association pamphlet gives this sample of two labels:

Brand A is acceptable:	Brand X is NOT acceptable:
"liquid safflower oil, partially hardened soybean oil, nonfat dry milk, etc."	"partially hydrogenated corn oil, liquid corn oil, nonfat dry milk, etc."

---

* This occasions much creative sneakiness by many manufacturers who arbitrarily declare their package to hold "2¾" servings or some such, thus reducing the number of the calories, grams of fat and sodium, etc., they have to display. Our favorite is a "no sugar" chocolate bar that proclaims two squares as "a serving," allowing them to list only 60 calories, a trap for the unwary.

Manufacturers who care more for sales than their customer's arteries try to fool you. You find "no cholesterol" or "made with 100% vegetable shortening" blazoned on the label of a product whose main ingredient is coconut or palm oil. Remember from chapter 3 that the cholesterol that clogs arteries is not the cholesterol one eats but cholesterol manufactured by the liver, which is stimulated to produce excess cholesterol by any saturated fat as much as by ingested cholesterol. Another label announces "pure vegetable oil," which turns out to be "partially hydrogenated," therefore saturated; still another boasts of being "high in polyunsaturates," when the product listing shows something like "specially processed vegetable oil" first, making that product even *higher* in saturated fats.

Your salvation is the mandated ingredients listing. Don't stop with the manufacturers' big-type blurbs; the truth, too often, is not in them. Read the ingredient listing; read the analysis if one is printed. And remember the magic words:

> hydrogenated
> hardened
> partially hardened or hydrogenated
> stabilized
> specially processed

Those are the words you don't want to see, except very near the end of any listing.

"Low fat" often presents another problem. A Heart Association newsletter points out that a certain brand of "low-fat" cheese contains about eight grams of fat per ounce, the amount found in two pats of butter. The only thing "low fat" means here is that this brand is lower in fat than most cheese, which is extraordinarily *high* in fat. Your only defense is to read the analysis to see how much fat "low fat" really is.

Our hero in these matters is Phil Sokolof, of Omaha, who in the late 1960s suffered a heart attack that he blamed on his 300 cholesterol count. Since then he has crusaded against manufacturers' wanton use of the so-called "tropical" oils, and saturated fats generally. He has forced some of the biggest manufacturers to back down. Our favorite Sokolof victory was his attack on Kellogg's Cracklin' Oat Bran, their attempt to cash in on the cholesterol-lowering fad for oat bran. It contained coconut oil! Kellogg first responded by calling Sokolof irresponsible, threatening to sue. Then they meekly allowed that, well, they'd find a way to eliminate the coconut oil. To date, Nabisco, General Mills, Pillsbury, Quaker Oats and seven other giants have also started to knuckle under.

You can help the process. When you see saturated fats listed, *especially* if one of those sneaky, deceptive blurbs enjoys prominence on the label, note the manufacturer, go the library, look up the manufacturer's corporate headquarters in Standard & Poor's corporate guide in the library, and write to the chief executive officer, with a copy to whoever is listed as VP of advertising or corporate communications. Say you'll stop buying *all* their products until they mend their ways, and you'll urge all your friends to join you. In fact, get some friends to sign it with you.

Sodium is a little harder to monitor than fat unless the label includes the complete analysis, listing actual quantities. Even so, you can infer the amount by noting where salt (or sodium in its various other forms) is listed among the ingredients. Just remember that anything with the word "sodium" in it counts—for example, "monosodium glutamate."

Of course, you can always write to ask a manufacturer who does not print an analysis exactly how much sodium is in any product.

Again, logic is the key.

Learn, What to and Where to

The family has to learn nutrition, and that is tough—because the health care profession, by and large, doesn't have a very good knowledge of nutrition. Nutrition is not well taught in medical schools, in my view. So you have to learn nutrition yourself, from books and articles and from those experts trained specifically in the field.

—Dr. Shahbudin Rahimtoola

You have to learn the principles behind the planning and preparation of balanced meals, plus the special techniques for reducing calories, fats, and sodium we discuss in this chapter and elsewhere in the book. It *is* tough, as Dr. Rahimtoola says, only because you cannot merely ask the doctor or nurse to tell you what you have to know. You must dig a little. The digging, though, is not that difficult. Here's some spade work.

First, a word of caution. The exact level of needed weight loss, calorie, fat, or sodium intake for your patient must come *only* from the attending doctor. They are not "nutrition." They are medical prescriptions. Nutrition is the art and science of how to achieve those and other commonly recognized goals of healthy eating. Doctors may not know much about the "means" (nutrition), but they are the only authority you should recognize for prescribing "ends."

As we suggested in chapter 7, "Going Home," you should seek an interview with the hospital dietitian or nutritionist. Failing that, you can probably find someone in the Yellow Pages listed under "nutritionist" (look there first) or "dietitian." The one you select should be either an M.D. or a registered dietitian (initials R.D. after the name). If you can find no one, write to the American Dietetic Association for names of those nearby (see p. 88).

For your own study we recommend the following pamphlets, which are available from The American Heart Association. Consult your local chapter.

"Nutritious Nibbles": A Guide to Healthy Snacking

"Nutrition for the Fitness Challenge"

"Nutrition Labeling" Food Selection Hints for Fat-Controlled Meals

"Recipes for Low-Fat, Low-Cholesterol Meals" (a selection from The *American Heart Association Cookbook*)

In addition, see the listings on page 112.

Moderation

A little egg yolk isn't going to kill anyone; a lot of fussing just conceivably might, and will certainly maim a relationship. "You shouldn't nag about every little lapse," says dietitian Sue Rogers. "'You mustn't eat this, you shouldn't eat that.' You're just swapping risk factors if diet becomes a source of stress and hostility and frustration."

Experienced people—doctors, families, patients themselves—agree.

I'll tell patients—this may sound like heresy—I'll tell them, If they want scrambled eggs for breakfast once a month, that probably isn't the end of the world. The consistent things a person does are more important. If they're out at a banquet and they serve roast beef, and it's the only time that month, no need to feel it's "guilt" or even "cheating."

—Dr. Frederick Grover

When they go back to the refrigerator and pick up cheese and this sort of thing, you have to learn not to nag. Because they're big boys, and they know.

—Mrs. J, patient's wife

The smartest thing a dietitian ever told me was, "If you get on a diet that is appropriate for you, and you make it a way of life, when you go to a banquet or out to a restaurant, occasionally, when it's an exception, you can do what you like."

> Don't make a pig of yourself; limit your quantities. But if what they have is mashed potatoes with gravy, have some mashed potatoes with gravy. Otherwise you're going to hate your diet and be miserable.
>
> —Mr. McI, a patient

Notice we're talking about lapses; "moderation" applies to them, strongly. If violation of the doctor's orders or nutritionist's suggestions becomes wholesale, intervention is essential. But make it a matter of conference, including the patient and the professional, not a matter of freelance nagging.

Out, Eating

Like much else discussed in these pages, eating out is a lot easier (and tastier) nowadays for those with coronary conditions. A more general awareness of low fat and low sodium pervades public consciousness and restaurant menus.

In many cities, restaurants mark dishes with a heart to signify their coronary acceptability. The American Heart Association has done a marvelous job of lobbying and education. Today, those on a severe sodium-restricted diet can ask restaurants to broil, grill, or fry their order without adding salt and be pretty sure of compliance. Many restaurants even promote low-sodium dishes.

In many places, the local Heart Association chapter provides a guide listing restaurants that purposively include dishes that (in the words of one local pamphlet) "meet the American Heart Association's standards for being low in fat and cholesterol, and may be lower in calories."

Still, under the best conditions, eating out can present a considerable problem. "You get guidance from a dietitian," says Mr. McI,

> then you report back and say, "I was doing OK but then this fellow took me to lunch. What do we do when go to lunch?"
>
> The dietitian says, "Choose only those things on the menu that will fit within your diet." Well, very rarely can you do this. I've tried, and you end up with toast and tea and a salad. And the dietitian says, "Well then that's what you do."
>
> But that is *not* what you do because somewhere along the line you must consider quality of life.

He complains with considerable justice about the evident unreality with which too many professionals view the world:

> They'll say, "You can have a taco—shredded lettuce, not much cheese, a little bit of lean ground meat." But that isn't the way any place makes tacos. Let them try to go out and eat in restaurants and stay on their diet following advice like that.

What does he do?

> When I go out, I prepare for it: the meal before and the meal after, I have nothing that has any calories to speak of.

Unfortunately, that incorporates its own unrealism: Mr. McI is highly self-disciplined, highly motivated; furthermore, he lives in a reasonably small community, works close to home, can mostly control and plan his occasions for eating out. For those less fortunate, perhaps less disciplined, the principles of hierarchical choice discussed above in "Fat" offer help. You prefer things broiled, roasted, or grilled rather than fried, prefer fried over deep fried; plain is better than with a sauce, a wine sauce is better than a cream sauce. You'd choose a lean London broil over a steak, but if you must have steak, you'd take sirloin (trimming away the visible fat) over filet mignon (whose fat is inextricably marbled into the meat); you'd choose veal over beef (but *not,* for instance, veal parmigiano—a fried or deep-fried cutlet layered with cheese—over roast beef), fish or chicken over veal, keeping in mind, again, the difference that variations in preparation can make (i.e., chicken à la king is no bargain in fat or calories).

Mashed potatoes seem a wiser choice than French fried, unless you add butter or they surround a lake of greasy gravy; a baked potato is better than either, but not soggy with butter or sour cream. If you must have butter on your vegetables, at least insist on putting it on yourself, in dollops, rather than letting them trowel it on in the kitchen. The same goes for bread. For salads, if you have the dressing on the side, you will surely put on less than the kitchen would; better yet, take Weight Watcher's tip and dip your fork vertically into the dressing, using for each bite only what sticks to the tines.

The guiding principle is to opt for those choices that minimize calorie/fat intake while sacrificing minimal satisfaction.

As we saw in "Fat," coronary common sense can reign even with fast foods. "There are better choices to make at fast food places, and there are worse choices," says dietitian Sue Rogers:

> Let's say you're used to grabbing a hamburger five nights a week because you're on the run and, come 6 o'clock, you're too hungry to wait for dinner at home.
>
> I'd start by giving some fast food information: "Look at how high in fat that is!"
>
> You say, "Wow! I didn't realize it was that high; I can order a fish sandwich." Then you check the charts and realize that's *still* pretty high in fat. So I'll say, "What can you order that's better that you can get

along with?" What you find, perhaps, is that the smallest cheeseburger is half the fat of what you used to order, and, yes, you can get along with that to kill your hunger until you get home.

You're still eating fast food five nights a week, but now you're making a better choice.

Better still, you might end up carrying a turkey sandwich with you in the car.

The logic of it is simple and easy to follow.

Own Program, Creating Your

If you're talking to a poor farmer from eastern Kentucky, you can say, "Go on a low-cholesterol diet." But if he grows cattle and hogs, there isn't much point in saying, "You can't have beef or ham."

Tell him to eat fish? Well, if it's summertime, maybe he can get fish; but if he's going to fry it in bacon fat, that doesn't do you any good.

All I'm saying is that you have to involve yourself enough with the patient and family to be able to treat them as individuals, not as part of some nutrition "program."

—Polly Brown

To be successful, every nutrition program must finally be your own, whether you are patient, spouse, or family member. Only the youngest children can be *required* to eat right; everyone else must sign on to a program or it simply won't work. "I guess my philosophy over time has become," says dietitian Sue Rogers, "instead of pushing them to eat what *we* consider the perfect diet, which they'll probably feel frustrated with the moment they walk out the door, I try to enlist their help in making that decision and *improving* their diet."

Consider Mr. McI. He has an engineering degree plus an MBA; he heads his own business. He says he wasn't smart enough to follow the convolutions of the diet programs offered him. "Both Frieda and I," he says,

found it very difficult to translate the instructions into ways of living— eating the exact right amount of the exact right food, a slice and a half of bread is equal to this, a teaspoon of butter is equal to that. I had that lecture, I guess, three times from three different dietitians. But no books, no lectures seemed to penetrate my thick skull.

I've talked to other people and they've had a similar experience. It appears that the only people who think this works are the dietitians and the doctors.

The problem is that everything is different. The amount of exercise you have a day is different, your routine is different, the amount of food you eat, whether you're eating out or eating at home, whether you eat at six o'clock or five o'clock, whether you take a walk with the dog or don't take a walk—all these things affect you. But the dietitians say, "Keep the same schedule; eat so many calories: You get a cup of coffee and two pieces of bread and a bowl of cereal with nonfat milk and sweetener on it and one apple for breakfast—and here are ways to convert that basic breakfast into dozens of others by using food exchanges."

It's like a great big puzzle. It has nothing to do with what's actually in the kitchen to eat that morning. Then a snack at 10 o'clock, two crackers and a piece of cheese, except if your cholesterol's high . . . My life isn't that regular. If I'm due to eat something at 10 o'clock, people come in, I can't do it. I'm due to have lunch with somebody tomorrow at one o'clock; then we go out to dinner, and I don't know what's going to be on the menu. I found it extremely difficult if not impossible to follow the instructions. Maybe it's my stubbornness.

More likely, he's unfortunate in the dietitians he encountered.

What does Mr. McI think should have happened? "They should have had me keep a record of what I actually eat for a few days or a week," he says, "then tinker with it, alter the diet one thing at a time. 'Can you live with this? Can you do this?'"

And what do experienced dietitians do?

"Before they come in for a nutrition consult," says Sue Rogers,

they fill out a three-day food history, exactly what they ate and drank and how much.

Let's say they're 20 pounds overweight. After we go through their diet history I might point out, "It's not the starchy food you're getting all the calories from, it's the fried fish; you're getting too much fat."

When I suggest some things, they say, "Gee! I didn't know that was a problem! I can give that up easy!" With others, they'll say, "No!" The dietitian makes suggestions, then patients have to decide how that fits in with their life and what they're going to do with that.

It should be small changes, incremental over time. We're talking eating habits that may go back 30, 50, 70 years, and to expect that they're going to eat the perfect diet tomorrow is ridiculous; making them try would be extremely stressful.

I encourage slow improvements. Let's say that they used to eat three strips of bacon every day; a great place to start would be, "Can you go to one strip? What a major decrease in fat intake! Work on that for a while, and then later think about cutting back even more."

It's exactly the advice Mr. McI was looking for. Since he didn't get it, he had to work things out for himself. "I just went off meat entirely," he says, just ate turkey and chicken and fish, and lots of vegetables; stayed off fat.

Seven years later, I've come to know what different kinds of food do to me. I jiggle it around depending on what I forecast my day will be like, then hope there will be no surprises.

I've gotten to a point—well, a week ago they said, "Your cholesterol is high; do you want to see the dietitian?" And I said, "No I know what to do." I know how to taper off on the food, and how to adjust my blood sugar—without having to measure.

Marry the two thoughts. As Sue Rogers puts it:

> If people learn the skills to evaluate what they're eating—not going by some canned pattern but by learning how to make choices and make decisions on how to eat—they're more likely to be successful in the long run.

Knowing about fats and sodium, what foods contain how much of what, knowing what cooking methods add or subtract what you don't want, knowing how certain foods affect particular people— knowing all this, plus the eating habits of your patient, yourself, the family (maybe all of you should keep a three-day or week-long food diary)—then you can "negotiate" (with them, with yourself) sensible, effective, comfortable changes.

If you have the help of a savvy dietitian, all the better. But the literature you need is always available from the Heart Association. It depends finally on the individuals involved anyway. All of you can do it together.

Salt/Sodium

"In my class," says dietitian Mary Bowlby, "I explain that sodium is an acquired taste and that when you take it away you miss it only initially. Then you get so that you can hardly stand much salt; it spoils food for you."

Unfortunately, the taste was acquired by humans a good many thousands of years ago,* and is very hard to shake off. Fortunately, we've acquired a taste for only one form: sodium chloride, salt. No one would sprinkle, say, sodium benzoate (or the other forms used as preservatives) on a steak or stalk of celery. So cutting down on

---

* Witness the antiquity of references: the Bible's "ye are the salt of the earth," and worries about salt losing its savor; the measure of people being "worth their salt" (from the days when it was a valuable spice), and those deemed inferior being at the far end of the table, "below the salt."

other forms of sodium is relatively easy, involving mostly inspection of all labels, plus a realization that certain food processes, such as curing meats (e.g., corned beef), involve sodium.

Control of salt intake is harder because we do indeed crave it on and in food. What to do?

The answer is, substitute other tastes—on a schedule that depends on how rigorous and abrupt the reduction must be. Patients with problems such as congestive heart failure have to cut out sodium intake almost totally and instantly. For others, the withdrawal can be gradual, the amount of salt used in cooking reduced as the level of other ingredients builds.

In either case, the object is to replace salt flavor with other acceptable flavors. A browse through Craig Claiborne's low-sodium cookbook ("Cookbooks," above) will give you the idea; American Heart Association pamphlets on use of herbs will give you specific pointers.

Some cases defeat substitution: nuts are either salted or not. But options always exist. If you like nuts, you may find you still like them well enough without salt; or you might substitute unsalted trailmix— a combination of nuts, raisins, and other goodies that, by combining tastes, leaves you oblivious to the missing salt.

Obviously, the rest of the family need not join in sodium reduction; they can add their own salt from the shaker. That may help if your patient's sodium reduction must be total and immediate, but it's a bad idea, long term. First, the less salt for everyone in the family, the better; it promotes hypertension in everyone, puts extra strain on every heart. Just as important, what your patient must do *is* a family matter, and all aspects of it should be treated as such. Besides, Mary Bowlby is right: we *can* lose this age old craving. "In my family," she says, "we're at the point now where at least one of my kids complains if we have ham for supper. Makes him thirsty."

Summing Up

A short after-dinner speech.

Some people are easy to cook for, others are difficult, with or without coronary conditions. The condition does not change that. Those who were pleased with family meals before can be just as pleased now. It may take a degree more care, attention, planning, thought, and work—but only a degree—with health benefits for the entire family rewarding the effort.

You have on your side the fact that everyone involved knows the reason for change. Attitude plays a major role. The whole family will greet "a heart-patient's diet" the way anyone takes to *any* diet, grudgingly; if, however, they're served "coronary cuisine"—imaginative, varied, well-prepared food that happens to be very healthy—they all will eat it right up!

Rehabilitation

Something I'd really like patients and families to be informed about is preventive maintenance.

A treatment, whether it's angioplasty or heart operation, really any treatment for coronary disease, is an intermediate step. It's extremely important that the patient and the family be educated and follow up for the long term to stop the progression of the disease or even reverse some of it.

—Dr. Allan Lansing
Louisville

That's a very important thing. Rehabilitation, in the broadest sense, is very, very critical.

—Dr. Lawrence Cohn
Boston

Almost everybody who's had a cardiac event could benefit by some aspect of cardiac rehabilitation.

—Dr. William Dafoe
Ottawa

Attitude

"We didn't do the surgery," one nurse tells patients, "so you can go home and be an invalid. It was to give you a meaningful lifestyle. There are things you can do to maintain that lifestyle for a longer period without significant heart problems." That, broadly, is rehab. Until *your* patient, your family and *you* all understand and buy into that concept, the best rehab program can't mean much, indeed may not do much good.

One patient, Mr. H, went with his wife to examine his hospital's rehab facility and suffered instant disenchantment. "It was a bad-smelling basement, all equipment and dials," he says.

> When Janice and I went down in this mustard-colored tile room, cold and empty with all the dials, and I was supposed to get on this bicycle and get wired up to a meter, and then pedal for 20 or 30 minutes, for some reason I said, "I'm not going to be a machine, I'm not going to do this." I walked off, and I didn't take the exercise program.

Another patient became depressed when told about rehab. "Where's it all going to end?" he wailed to a visitor. "I had a heart attack, I've had heart surgery, now they tell me I need to go to cardiac rehab? What's next?"

In the first place, rehab means more than stationary bicycles and monitors; exercise is central to the concept but by no means all.* Pam Moore, nurse manager of a Los Angeles hospital rehab center, calls it a "multi-functional group," combining exercise that progressively (and safely, because of those monitors) taxes the heart with increasing demands, nutritional guidance, and lifestyle changes such as lessons in stress management. All comes in the context of mutual support, with patients learning from other patients, comparing notes and experiences. "Where does it end? What's next?" It never ends (although formal, regular attendance at rehab generally stops after six weeks or a few months) because what's next is a lifelong commitment to doing what enhances lifestyle and prolongs life.

To get started—which is all that formal rehab is, a guided start—requires just one thing: "We ask people to make a commitment," says Dr. Dafoe of his program,

> both in terms of compliance and some of the things they're going to be working on. If people are not motivated, if they attend episodically, we have them go off the program because there are so many well-motivated people wanting to be on the program.

Commitment is the essence of the right attitude.

---

* The patient who walked away from rehab continued walking—for exercise. Perhaps significantly, he experienced a difficult recovery with severe psychological problems. Ironically, he fully perceives the need for exactly the sort of holistic support group he might have found at rehab, assuming that his hospital offered the right kind of program, and he regrets not having had its benefit.

Effectiveness

Most programs start about three weeks after the patient has returned home, when, studies show, patients are ready to listen and ready to make necessary lifestyle changes and commitments. "People come to rehab in a wheelchair," says Carole Landers.

> They have made themselves, or their families have made them, invalids. It amazes me to see them turn around when you start talking to them about their risk factors and their goals, even if the goal is only to go out and play a game of golf.

Rehab works, but not automatically. Without effort and commitment, without the changes that rehab seeks to effect, says Albert McClure, "we've seen patients return within five years, or even two years or three years, for a second surgery. . . . I have no trouble at all motivating those: two surgeries are enough to motivate anybody."

The president of Humana's Mended Hearts chapter visited a 35-year-old who was back for a second bypass after four years. "You won't see me back here in four more years," said the chastened re-op. "I'm going to listen this time."

Family, Role of the

> Support from the family, especially the spouse, is one of the major factors; if the spouse is not supportive then it's very hard.

> —Marja-Leena Keast
> Physiotherapist

> A lot of times the patient won't be as receptive in the beginning as the family will. So they have to support the patient by saying, "Yes, let's go on in to rehab." And the patient will start responding. The role of the family in support is a must. You must have that support.

> —Carole Landers
> Rehab Nurse Manager

In rehab, the basic rule for families is the same as for doctors in their practice: "First, do no harm." Professionals note, with fear, the tendency of some families to be overly protective, discouraging patients from exerting themselves. Rehab people want patients to be as physically active as they safely can.

What can the family do to help? "Make sure the patient participates," says one doctor. As the two quotes that start this entry suggest, that role is vital.

The best rehab programs are holistic (see "How Rehab Works," below), covering even behavior modification as it applies to such matters as eating, stress, and smoking. But the most obvious and immediate aspect of rehab is the physical conditioning that anybody who has undergone the trauma of coronary occlusion or surgery (or both) needs in order to regain full function. Patients often don't feel like exercising. They may hurt; the exercise may hurt; fears may assail them: "Can my heart take the strain?" The tendency often, at first, is to grump in bed, the wrong thing.

"Don't let them just sit there and sulk," says John Snyder, himself once a patient, now president of his Louisville Mended Hearts Chapter. "Some patients do. I've been called at home by the wives of some patients I've visited. The wife will say, 'He's sitting here crying because he hurts and he doesn't trust himself, now that he's out of the hospital.'"

Snyder sympathizes, because he did much the same. "In my case," he says,

> first couple of days, yes, I wanted to stay in bed.
>
> In the hospital, the nurses took us up and down the steps a couple of times, and walked us around the halls. So my wife said, "Let's get out of bed and do some walking like we did in the hospital."
>
> And then she said, "Let's go up and down the stairs." So I said, "Yes! That sounds like a good idea."

"Like we did in the hospital" was the master stroke: it recalled him to what he knew he should be doing, and relieved his fears of overdoing; if it was all right then, right after surgery, it had to be all right now, 10 or more days later.

This period, before any formal rehab, is crucial. As Snyder puts it, "after you get home until you go back to the cardiac rehab center, that's when the family has to encourage the individual to start walking—so you can get the heart pumping, and doing things—not just sit there and vegetate." The process is so crucial, another wife calls this the only real justification she can think of for nagging. That's true from the beginning, and continues to be true. "It's very important," she says, "and they tend not to want to do this after they get home. When he starts complaining about his legs aching, I just can't keep from saying, 'But you haven't been *walking*. You should be walking at least three days a week.'"

That's where the entire family comes in. As you'll see, below, some patients have their exercise monitored long distance, by telephone hookup to the rehab center. Pam Moore, a rehab nurse manager in Los Angeles, prefers to avoid that whenever possible. "You need," she says, "the psychological group support of other people. When you're riding a bike hooked up to a telephone, you're isolated." At very least, she says,

. . . from the start, it should be a family process. The kids go out walking, too. And if the patient, at first, can only walk around the dining room table, that's great! It's individualized, not some competition. The kids join in and everybody's involved. It's going to bring the family closer together.

For the long haul, family support for the holistic package of rehab is equally crucial, albeit less dramatic, which of course is the problem. "It's forever," says one doctor. "You can get 'up' for something very dramatic in your life. But the further you get out from the event, the less important is seems." So family support must be sustained; exercise, right eating, stress reduction, the works, all must become a family habit.

But what's so bad about that?

How Rehab Works

One of the themes we see in this program is that everything is interrelated.

—Dr. William Dafoe

Details vary, but enough congruence exists among the rehab programs at five hospitals we visited from Ottawa to Santa Monica that we're confident the following represents a standard for comprehensive programs at good hospitals.

Typically, the program starts two or three weeks after discharge from the hospital* with a painstaking evaluation of the patient (the spouse usually in attendance), including a medical examination to assess the proper starting level of exercise for each patient.

A rehab professional, often a specially trained nurse, walks patient and spouse through the facts about risk factors and how to mitigate them, assessing the risks inherent in the patient's vocation. The nurse generally makes appointments for the patient and spouse to see a nutritionist, and sometimes a stress-management counselor. If any family issues surface, a social worker may intervene.

Formal exercise sessions start with the patient monitored one-on-one by a rehab specialist to make sure the patient's heart easily tolerates the amount of exercise being done. These sessions typically last about an hour, and occur once or twice a week for about three weeks. Meanwhile the patient starts home exercise, a combination of prescribed, light, aerobic calisthenics and measured walking. Classes

---

* Some participants are angina sufferers who have never been in the hospital.

or interviews for the long-term molding of lifestyle in nutrition continue.

The next phase finds the patient, perhaps still monitored, but no longer with such an eagle-eye, exercising in a group of three or four, usually three times a week.

After evaluation, some centers provide monitoring by telephone for patients who live too far away from the center for reasonable commuting. Patients exercise while hooked up to measuring devices that send signals by telephone, again allowing safe, progressive increases in the demands exercise puts on the body and heart as exercise makes both grow stronger. Except for the reservation expressed by the rehab nurse in the entry above—that patients need interaction with other patients during this phase—such monitoring works well.

Like any muscle, the heart gains strength with exercise that pushes it beyond normal activity. The heart's only exercise is the contraction we call "beating." So to strengthen your heart, you must set it beating faster than it goes normally, normal being called the "resting heart rate," somewhere between 60 and 90 beats a minute. You ascertain your resting heart rate by taking your pulse after sitting quietly for five minutes or so. The object is to exercise enough so that the heart rate increases by at least ten beats a minute (anywhere up to 30 beats a minute is fine), always with the stipulation that it should never exceed a rate equal to 200 minus your age. If you are 40, you should never push your heart rate beyond 160 (200–40 = 160); if you are 63, 137 is maximum (200–63 = 137).

With a resting heart rate of 78, to strengthen your heart you must exercise long and hard enough to boost your rate (pulse) to at least 88 (the higher the better, up to 108) and keep it there for 20 minutes. Plainly, as you get generally stronger, that takes more and more exercise.

The instruction sheet one hospital gives patients assumes this progression: the first week you walk on a level, paved surface about one-quarter mile, with hospital-taught, aerobic arm and leg exercises repeated ten times, twice a day; by the fourth week you're walking one mile on a level surface, with 25 repetitions of the exercises. In the seventh week, the surface includes hills and rough terrain—twice as much exercise as on a level paved surface—with the distance cut back to a half mile. By week 12, you walk four miles a day and you deliberately climb stairs (three times as hard as walking on level surfaces) as often as you can, comfortably. From there on, say the instructions, "Continue to do your walking four miles every day the rest of your life"—with the indulgence that the four miles can be broken into mile-plus chunks as you will. For inclement weather, the instructions suggest places such as shopping malls, school gym tracks, grocery store aisles, stationary bikes, and treadmills.

Can the patient overdo it? Checking is easy. Remember that the exercise should elevate the heart rate 10–30 beats a minute for 20 minutes. After exercise, the patient rests, sitting, for five minutes. The pulse should be no faster than five beats a minute more than it was before exercise started. If it is, you cut back the amount of exercise until the pulse returns to within that five-beat limit.

The combination of rehab center exercise, lifestyle consultations, and home exercise is well calculated to put any patient (and family!) on the way to excellent long-term recovery and long-term, high-quality living.

Own Program, Your

Suppose your hospital doesn't offer a rehab program, or has only a program so rudimentary or in such unappetizing surroundings that, like Mr. H in "Attitude," above, your patient is instantly turned off and refuses to participate. Mr. H, as noted, constructed his own exercise program, followed it conscientiously, and did well with it.

Only two things disqualify that as a pattern for others. First, Mr. H had received bypass surgery before any infarction had a chance to damage his heart, so strain on the heart hardly counted as a consideration. Second, although the exercise part of rehabilitation was fine, the rest of Mr. H's accommodation to a new lifestyle, without professional guidance, was forbiddingly rocky.

How, instead, should your family proceed? "I think," says Carole Landers,

> you *have to have a physician* at the beginning, to evaluate the patient, set levels of exercise, and try to instill the importance of exercise and of changing risk factors.
>
> Certainly the family needs to be brought in each time the physician talks to that patient.
>
> We have a good example in the southern part of the state—a small, 43-bed hospital that does an excellent job, although it does not have a cardiac rehab unit.
>
> For their heart patients, they have devised a calisthenics program for home, and a walking or bicycle program. They keep in touch by volunteers calling and asking patients how they're doing.
>
> About once a month they have meetings where they do health teaching, talking about risk factors.
>
> So there's always a way.

Sure, you say, but they're a hospital.

Not really; not for these purposes. They perform the much simpler function, not of provider of services, but only of procuring and coordinating the services of others. That is a function the family can provide equally well.

Your own program *must* start by insisting, as Landers does, on an attending physician's evaluation of the patient's condition, then prescription of progressive exercise limits and goals. How far can the patient walk the first time out of bed? the first week? first month? How about lifting things such as children? groceries? When? how heavy? How soon can the patient resume golf? sex? washing the car? mowing the lawn? Arranging such talks should present little problem; chances are the surgeon or cardiologist or both will *insist* on such discussions. (If they refuse to discuss the subject, review "Doctors, Switching" in chapter 6.)

With that base, you can arrange to see a nutritionist and a physical therapist. If neither doctor nor hospital can refer you to such specialists, they are listed (under those headings) in the Yellow Pages.

Support groups are another resource. Most hospitals have so-called "zipper clubs" or Mended Hearts chapters. But you can organize your own group with the patients (and families) you encounter at the hospital. You're all in the same boat; pull together.

From there, the only problems are those faced by families with access to the best rehab programs imaginable: keeping up the patient's motivation to attend and comply. But those problems, which we examine throughout this chapter, are no more severe. As Carole Landers says, there's always a way.

Risks

What we do in rehabilitation is not entirely risk-free. But the risks are very low, the benefits enormous!

—Dr. William Dafoe

The risk, however low a number you assign it, constitutes the compelling reason for having exercise programs designed and supervised by trained physical therapists, working within a doctor's prescribed limits for *this* patient, and at least toward the beginning, electronically monitoring the heart's reaction to the exercise. The details mean nothing: whether it's a rehab center therapist or one you select for your own program; whether the monitor is in the same room or a telephone line away. The point is to have this aspect of rehab be professional. That's because exercise, in terms of rehab, is not what you may imagine. Playing golf three times a week may be fun, but it won't strengthen your heart appreciably unless you walk the 18 holes, carrying your own bag, which brings up some problems, at least in the beginning. Lifting weights not only won't do much for your heart, it constricts blood vessels and could cause problems. "There are *safe* ways to exercise," says Carole Landers,

> and cardiac patients need to learn the safe ways.
> There are effective ways to exercise that they need to learn, too. Like knowing they should be exercising seven minutes and achieving *this* heart rate versus just going out and doing whatever they think is good.
> You'd be surprised what they think is exercise! If you asked 10 people, eight would tell you different things. And most would be wrong, especially when we talk about heart disease.

No, we're not going to delve into the safe ways here, any more than we would dream of prescribing medicine. We said this subject required professionals, which we are not. See a physical therapist, after you've talked about it with a doctor.

We can tell you about METs, metabolic equivalents, which are a measure of how much energy you expend in a given activity. One MET is the energy it takes to sit quietly in a chair, hands in lap, feet on the floor. What points the way to safe exercise is that many activities demand fewer METs than you would suppose. For instance, chopping wood takes 10 METs; sawing wood requires only 4–5. And for that same expenditure of energy you could go dancing, walk at the good clip of 3.5 mph, or play golf, carrying your own clubs. Women will find an odd comfort (and perhaps ammunition) in the fact that stripping a bed takes 1–2 METs *more* than any of those, and is equivalent to lifting and carrying a 50-pound load.

The marvelous news is that sex takes no more METs than does light woodworking or attending church! (But see footnote on page 164.)

Who Needs Rehab and Why

Two views that appear contradictory:

> Ultimately, I think almost everybody who's had a cardiac event could benefit by some aspect of cardiac rehabilitation.
>
> —Dr. William Dafoe

> It's my contention that most people don't need a lot of rehabilitation after routine bypass surgery.
> If they're very sick and debilitated, then it's necessary. But it can be awfully expensive to go into a two-month rehabilitation when all you

need to do is get out and walk. And go back to work. So I think that one can overemphasize these rehabilitation programs.

The key to success with most people is to get them back to doing what they're used to doing, once they're over their aches and pains.

I refer patients to rehabilitation programs if I think they have problems, if they need that organized and structured support. But we try to instill enough confidence in the patients so they realize that once they get over the aches and pains, and have a stress test that looks better than it did when they started, they can go back and engage in their usual occupations.

—Dr. John Hutchinson

On analysis, there is less contradiction than might appear. No doctor questions the need for rehabilitation after surgery or the trauma of infarction or even the debilities of chronic angina. Some quarrel only with the need for *formal* rehab programs. A third opinion blends the two positions:

The level to which one should push oneself and the need for a rehabilitation program really depend on the individual patient: many have the internal discipline, combined with the family support, to build up an exercise program on their own. They don't need to be in a program.

Other patients, because of fear, or because of lack of extensive exercise in the past, definitely do need a rehabilitation program in order to get themselves to the correct level.

—Dr. Hillel Laks

Like Hutchinson, Laks also specifies that those who start their recovery very sick or debilitated *absolutely* need rehab programs for safety's sake, for the available monitoring and repeated stress testing.

For most, the question comes down to a matter of determination and willpower, being a "good patient." Hutchinson and Laks are plainly right that those who will exercise on their own don't "need" formal rehab programs; after all, a lot of people (including our husbands) made splendid, determined, complete rehabilitations before formal programs existed. But we've heard often enough from enough patients and families how much harder it is to do it on your own—both the exercise part and the knowledge-gathering for the necessary lifestyle changes—that we are inclined to believe that formal programs, even of the family's own devising, make a lot of sense.

One further note on who needs formal programs, again from Dr. Laks:

Rehabilitation programs and family support are much more critical in older patients. Under the age of 70, recovery is usually fairly standard and predictable. Above that, you need a tremendous amount of effort to make sure they don't lose what they had before the operation.

Rehabilitation programs, family support, friends, outside interests—they all become very critical.

Those patients should be in a rehabilitation program where they have the discipline of having to exercise on a regular basis, with a secondary program worked out, usually with the help of a spouse, for activities such as visiting friends, going out to dinner, hobbies, going to the theater, etc., regardless of whether they "feel like" those activities or not. Because without that discipline, they could easily regress and lose interest in life. And you then get a vicious cycle of depression and less and less involvement.

That age group is a great challenge. It really takes a concerted effort to get that group of patients through the operation and fully rehabilitated to the point where they can enjoy life as much or more than before.

With all age groups, the family can help meet the challenge.

CHAPTER 12

Children

Attitude
Problems Related to the Heart Condition
Problems, Unrelated
Whole Family Involved

Attitude

You always knew you'd have problems with your children. Not because of anyone's heart condition; that just changes a few forms the problems take. You have children; they have problems and give you some; long ago you decided that the problems of having children were well worth the rewards.

What you know as a parent is not suddenly obsolete because you are, now, also the spouse of someone with a heart condition. Sometimes the spouse must overrule the parent—as in mandating lifestyle changes for the entire family, or in forbidding undue hullabaloo when your patient needs rest. That does not mean your judgment as a parent is wrong, just that it has been temporarily displaced or modified by circumstance. It is simply a matter of priorities.

Just remember the continuing needs of children. That should offset the sheer novelty of your other, newer role. You have been a parent longer; you take that function in stride. You have not gotten the hang of being the spouse of someone with a heart condition, so everything connected with that role seems momentous. The danger is that you may overestimate the importance of what you do as "coronary spouse" compared with what you do as parent. Even when the children's activities or problems bear no discernible relation to your spouse's heart problems, you may start to judge them in that light, which can make them seem trivial and therefore dismissible, not requiring attention unless they might conceivably contribute to . . . The Problem. This can translate as something on the order of "No, you may not

154

try out for the football team: the worry about your getting hurt could *kill* your mother!" Or, "No you may not complain about the creepy way your little sister is behaving; it disturbs your father to hear you fight."

What you are really saying, both to yourself and, worse, to your children, is that they no longer have problems, that no one does, really, except the patient. Such notions can result in tragedy. Mr. Y had been unusually close to his 15-year-old son. "They would go camping with the Boy Scouts, everything!" Mrs. Y told us. "They had a great relationship." Then came Mr. Y's heart attack—while, in fact, the son was away at camp. He called, wanting to come home; Mrs. Y, feeling that her own problems, worries, and needs had to be almost totally repressed for fear they might affect her husband, felt it best not to import a possible extra set of problems, worries, and needs, so said no, the boy should stay at camp until his father was back from the hospital and on the way to recovery. "From that point on," Mrs Y told us,

> their whole relationship was different. He was terrified that if he upset his father in any way, he might cause him to have another heart attack.
>
> Seeing that look on his face years later, when his father would come home at night, and the first thing he'd say was, "How do you feel?"— it's so wrong! . . .
>
> I really felt very unhappy for him because I realized that it wasn't a normal growing-up situation. He thought, before he did anything, what his father's reaction might be and if it might endanger his health. That's not very wholesome.

At the time we spoke with Mrs. Y, the son, at age 25, remained the same; he had never gotten over his fear that he might somehow precipitate another heart attack; the relationship had never returned to normal.

Another teenager developed symptoms of his own heart condition. When all possible tests demonstrated that nothing was physically wrong, the parents turned to a psychiatrist for help, and it soon became clear that his mother's almost total attention to her husband's health had made the boy terribly jealous, his subconscious conspiring with his body to produce the thing that his emotions recognized as the most "effective" way to get attention: a heart condition just like Dad's, the one that wins Mom's attention.

What can you do about all this? Dislocations *will* distort your children's lives; in some measure, their wants *will* be subordinated to a patient's needs; they *will* receive somewhat less of both parents' absorbed attention, certainly at first. In the case of the boy who had developed a psychosomatic heart condition, the psychiatrist helped him understand that his mother's sudden shift of "interest" from him to his father had nothing to do with love but with a real physical need on his father's part. Incredibly, no one had bothered to help the boy think through what any human being in his mother's position must be feeling and fearing, or what the sure results of those emotions must be. When he did know, the boy had little trouble grasping the fact that his mother did not love him less, but that she was reacting, herself, to his father's immediate and important need.

Your children will be the same. Just make sure they understand that none of the dislocations in their lives because of the heart condition has a thing to do with the love that either of you feel for them. When they were babies, their needs, being more urgent, came before your needs; now, sometimes, it's the other way around, and for the same reason: it has nothing to do with love, only with relative physical need.

If you continue to see your children's needs as valid claims even when you must subordinate them to the more urgent needs of a heart patient, you will almost automatically arrange to do it without making the children ever feel they are any less loved and needed by either parent.

Problems Related to the Heart Condition

We examined the basic heart-related problem in "Attitude," above: the necessary diminution of sheer attention you and your patient may have to pay to the children for a while. The solution is simply making the children understand why your preoccupation is necessary and why it signifies no change at all in how much they're loved and needed.

Explanation, full and frank, also solves the possible problem of the effect that any personality change, however temporary (see chapter 9), may have on the children. First, they should understand the possibility that a loving parent may suddenly and inexplicably seem _____ (select a word appropriate to the age and understanding of the children: cranky, hostile, upset, fringe-paranoid, or whatever), but tell them ahead of time what to expect and (more or less, again depending on age and understanding) why, so they don't think it's capricious or personal. They must understand that whatever the contrary evidence of their senses (and momentarily hurt feelings), this once and future loving parent does not suddenly hate them or, worst of all, hold them responsible for the heart condition.

That's essential. Mr. F specifies that both he and his wife, during her nine-year struggle with arrhythmia and congestive heart failure, before a successful transplant, took pains repeatedly to "make clear to the children that this was no one's fault, no one *caused* anything to happen, this is simply what *is*."

Notice the words "no one's fault." Make it clear that includes the patient. After all, you don't want the children "blaming" any unavoidable family dislocations on the person with the heart condition any more than you want them blaming themselves.

Remember in all this that a sense of perspective and moderation is most useful. For instance, your patient must get more than usual rest at first, so needs more than usual quiet. But it is not all-or-nothing. One disturbed nap, one hour less of rest, one upset, one tumult—or two or three, for that matter—is not the end of the world or of the patient. If your children steal an hour's sleep, it is barely petty larceny, and no one's best interest is served by turning that into a "federal case."

Problems, Unrelated

Of course, your children will continue to have the same normal growing-up problems they had before the heart condition, and would have had without the condition. These problems bulk no more serious (but, alas, no less serious) than before. If you are satisfied that you generally handle them pretty well, keep doing whatever you have always done. Problems that have no connection with the heart attack should be kept that way.

Whole Family Involved

The surest way to eliminate problems with the children about the heart condition is (as it usually is) to enlist their support in eliminating problems. Children need to feel needed. Make them feel that, and they almost automatically feel loved. So rather than exacting compliance with any lifestyle changes you want to make, strive to get the children on your side, which is where their natural sentiment and affections encourage them to be, anyway. Angle your discussion toward the idea of "what you can do to help," and you make them part of the recovery process and proud of themselves for having an important role in what is clearly a matter of first importance for the family. Polly Brown puts it this way:

> Children's motivation cannot just be that they're scared something is going to happen to Mom or Dad; rather that they can take good care of themselves, and be part of grown-up decisions.

That slant helps disguise the fact that much of what the children can do to help may appear unsatisfyingly negative: *not* smoking, *not* raising too much ruckus, *not* complaining about the sudden lack of French fries and fried chicken, with a concurrent appearance of fish and abundance of herb- (rather than butter-) flavored vegetables, etc.

Instead, they become positive partners in sensible, healthy living for the entire family. One woman told us that her children rapidly became such convinced converts that "they've gotten, well, intolerant. If they see their father eating the wrong things, they'll say, 'Now you know you're just heading for another heart attack!'"

Beyond making them partners in the decisions, you can generally convince children that doing nothing is important if you turn it around to make something of nothing. Present them with a course of action that appears positive. For example, one woman had accompanied her husband on a business trip, on which he had a heart attack. She feared a bad effect on her husband if anyone were to make a dramatic cross-country trip to his bedside (they lived outside San Francisco, and he was in a Boston hospital). The only probable long-distance visitors were her mother-in-law, who lived with them and, while not an invalid, did need some attention, and their 17-year-old son, for whom she turned the negative "No, you cannot come," into a positive "Here's how you can help":

> He wanted to come—but I said, "No, I need you there. I'll need you there to help with Grandma. To keep her from worrying or trying to come, which would be too much for her."

Modest ingenuity will guide you to alternatives: taking care of younger children, enlisting them in the family's lifestyle changes, that sort of thing. If you are then appropriately lavish with your praise for the children's help, even those ways that seem objectively inconsequential take on gratifying importance. You will be pleased and proud of, and touched by, the maturity, consideration, and affectionate concern your children display, the way they rise to the occasion.

CHAPTER 13

Sex

Angina,	Effect of Heart Conditions	Impotence
Effect of	Physiologic	Satyriasis
	Psychologic	What to Do

We've all come to a more relaxed acceptance of our sexuality in the decade and a half since *Survive* was published.

And physicians, specifically, are much less restrictive now. We are apt to suggest more rapid resumption of sex after a myocardial infarction or any of the interventions—which perhaps makes it a little less frightening to the couple. If you have to wait six weeks, it's sort of like bike riding: you don't forget how to do it but it makes it a much more monumental event when you resume it.

So I think that with the very brief lull we have, and the assurance that there isn't going to be a major calamity, and without a lot of the restrictions and rigmarole and suggestions for this and that that we used to make, it in many instances is not a problem.

—Dr. Warren Goldburgh

This chapter, of course, is for the other instances—in the hope it can help add to those instances where sex is not a post-coronary problem or where the problems diminish rapidly.

Angina,* Effect of

The best exposition of this phenomenon comes from Polly Brown, who speaks with the authority of experience both as a working R.N.

---

* Properly speaking, this belongs with the entry below on the physiologic effects of coronary conditions on sex. Except, as you'll see, it also belongs in the entry on the psychologic effects. On the other hand, if we assume that surgery or medical treatment has eliminated angina, it has ceased to present a problem, so has no place at all in the chapter—save, perhaps, as a promise of relief for readers still awaiting treatment. In fact, we include it as a reminder that the physiologic-psychologic effects of coronary conditions on sex form a continuum, and that relief is not only possible but probable.

and a director of clinical coordinators, intimately involved in even more cases. She says,

> It's very common for a man with undiagnosed heart disease—during sex or getting ready for sex—to have angina. He doesn't know what it is, he just feels uncomfortable; so he becomes less affectionate and finally less responsive without telling her why. She thinks it's something she's done wrong.
>
> Why won't he discuss it with her? Until a doctor diagnoses his condition, he would never discuss it because he doesn't want her to know that he may have the kind of pain where he couldn't make love to her. That's the worst thing that could happen to a man. He won't discuss it even with his doctor!
>
> So when a patient has had several heart attacks, I sometimes bring up the subject with the couple very early, before surgery. I say there may have been, in their relationship, a problem with sex because of angina.
>
> Lo and behold, the man says, "Well, yes there has been a problem." And I say, "Well, that's another very good reason for going ahead and getting your heart fixed."
>
> If nobody brings up that topic with them, they both may just go along thinking, "Well, there's just something wrong with me." And that can destroy that whole part of their life together.

You can see the direct effect of the physiology of heart disease on the psychology of sex. And you can see that the twin solutions are medical treatment and ventilation of the problem.

Effect of Heart Conditions, Physiologic

With two exceptions, one of them only indirect, a heart condition that doctors have successfully treated has *no* effect on anyone's ability to have and enjoy sex.

Both exceptions apply only to men.

First, if the blood supply is restricted enough, as in congestive heart failure, there may not be enough blood flow to sustain an erection.

Second, medications that doctors use often cause at least temporary impotence. "A large percentage," says Dr. Goldburgh, "have some dysfunction after surgery, after infarction, and after almost anything except angioplasty. If I run into it, I feel I've done it with medicines, because of the number and the kind of drugs that we use; even if you don't have a problem we can give it to you." And, he hastens to add, doctors can generally take it away again, adjusting medication or doses.

The physiologic effect of sex on the heart is what scientists call "counterintuitive." You intuitively expect that the pounding heart, the heavy breathing, the perspiration are signs that the body, specifically heart and lungs, is undergoing a fierce workout. The conclusion seems obvious. As one wife put it,

> . . . I wasn't exactly frightened, but I thought, "Sex is one thing he's going to *feel!*" They put everything into it, you're using every muscle in your body. Your heart is pounding—and you can't help thinking, "What's going to happen?"

Nothing bad—unless your apprehension causes either or both of you to ruin the moment. What "common sense" tells you about the strain of sex on the heart is simply wrong. As we pointed out in chapter 11, "Risks," marital sex* requires the same energy output as light woodworking or attending church (or, to be sure, the theater). For anyone who's recovered sufficiently to return home and to be given the go-ahead by a doctor, sex is not only *not* dangerous, it counts as good aerobic exercise!

Significantly, the UCLA manual for transplant patients specifies that the only restrictions are on positions or athletics that cause pain, stress, or strain across the surgical incision, and that only for six weeks. The manual concludes, "After six weeks, no restrictions exist."†

Effect of Heart Conditions, Psychologic

This can differ markedly from the trivial physiologic effect of sex on the heart. Again, the effect is on men, not women, except in extreme cases where a refusal to listen to the facts about the coronary effect of sex generates enough fear to trigger frigidity.

Many years ago we examined the subject with Reuben Koller, Ph.D., a psychologist who specializes in the sexual problems of heart patients. Although that was many years ago, nothing has changed; his observations remain valid. He called the psychologic effect of a heart condition on sex "a spiral of impotence." While still in the hospital, immediately following infarction or surgery, a patient truly cannot have sex. His body, hurt, has no interest in it; his mind does not even bother with sexual fantasies; medications have very likely rendered him temporarily impotent anyway. But that normal condition passes soon. Indeed, in the days when coronary patients languished

---

* There is a point to specifying "marital," and a couple of tiresome jokes to go with it, that we examine in "What to Do," below.

† That by no means automatically applies to you and yours; certainly not in contravention of your doctor's orders. Remember, transplant recipients do not have damaged or repaired or reconditioned hearts; they have brand new, young ones.

in hospital for weeks, Dr. Koller told us, it was "not uncommon for a patient to have erections during certain activities, like when a nurse bathes him. . . ."

Today he's more likely to be home by the time the effects of coronary, surgical, and medicinal trauma have ended. That means he's gone home temporarily impotent. Even while giving permission to resume sex, the doctor has necessarily warned against undue strain (see the entry above). Some men will translate that injunction into fear of sex, a fear that his wife will make unfulfillable sexual demands on him, often linking it, as Dr. Koller pointed out, to other natural anxieties over the future. Psychologists call this "performance anxiety."

That starts the spiral. As Dr. Koller put it,

> Impotence is usually based on something like that. "I'm not going to be able to make it. Will she hate me when she realizes I can't do it? What'll happen to me—I'll be such a bad person, a failure." And all this stuff makes him fulfill his greatest fear. He's *not* able to do it *because* he's anxious. . . .
>
> . . . [Anxiety] could very easily lead to impotence. The part of the nervous system that deals with anxiety has to be shut down for sexual arousal to take place. An erection involves the part of the nervous system that is involved in sleeping. So if you're anxious, it's extremely difficult to get an erection. That's just the way our bodies are built. . . .
>
> Then the next time, you're more frightened, more anxious. And the next time, of course, you don't get your erection, either.

The spiral continues, today's anxiety causing today's impotence, which practically guarantees tomorrow's even greater anxiety, which causes . . . and so on. Long after the least physiologic problem has disappeared, the mind's erroneous perception of sex's effect on the heart can make it, at worst, somewhere between difficult and impossible, and, at best, decidedly unenjoyable for both partners.

Impotence

Briefly, reduced blood supply and medications can physically cause impotence; misplaced anxiety about "overexertion" and over fancied inability to perform can mentally cause it.

The most extreme example we know of psychologic impotence happened back when patients stayed in the hospital for weeks, well past the time when, physically, men were again ready and interested in sex. One woman told us,

> The doctor had said something about "no sex for a while" when he was still in the hospital. And he was scared of his reaction.

I went in to see him one day, and I put my hand under the blanket
and touched him—as a joke. And he said, "Don't do that, for God's
sake!"
He really was nervous about that. "Don't do that, God! Don't do
that!"

You can imagine how carefree and normal their sex life figured to
be once they got home. Through misunderstanding of the doctor's
temporary prohibition, the man's mind practically begged his body
to be impotent.

Satyriasis

This is the most benign of the sexual derangements, being self-
limiting, self-correcting, and even while it lasts reasonably inoffensive
(if sometimes fatiguing) in its progress.
One wife explained the condition this way:

I was very frustrated with the sexual situation for a reason I didn't
expect. My husband seemed to be more interested than usual. He was
trying to prove something to himself, and I didn't know how to handle
that situation.

I went to talk to the doctor, but he just sort of tossed it off casually.
And I guess I decided, well, the doctor wasn't that concerned, so I must
be wrong to be worried.

Anyway, things just got back to normal by themselves. We got back
into our old patterns and that was that. It was a temporary thing.

Another woman called her husband's attitude about sex, once the
doctor said it was all right to resume intercourse, "uncontrollable,"
insisting on sex every night, whereas before it had been only when,
as she said, "the spirit moved them." She also felt her husband seemed
to be proving himself—to her as much as to himself: he kept asking
her during, immediately after, and between times, whether she enjoyed
sex as much as before. It also seemed tied to her husband's insistence
on returning to the same work he had been doing before the attack,
which involved more physical labor than she thought good for him.

Not knowing what to do, she did nothing. Yet, within six months
their sex life had returned to normal. And he had changed jobs.

Both patterns are classic. Men often wonder, at various age mile-
stones, how "potent" they still are in every sense, including sexual. A
heart condition outpaces any birthday in making a man anxious
about such matters. "In my experience," Dr. Koller told us,

that stops of its own accord, especially if he's given some support, if
he's treated normally, not like an invalid. He's trying to see how

attractive he is, particularly to his wife. It is not a sign that he's going to be adulterous.

Actually, this satyriasis is almost the opposite of adultery. What the man is trying to prove to himself and to his wife is best proved in bed with her, not in clandestine motels. Which is why the condition cures itself. As we've stressed elsewhere, sex is not burdensome on the heart; the heart condition itself in no way impedes sexual performance. Once the satyr finds that out, he no longer has to prove anything. His interest in sex, for better or worse, quickly subsides to whatever level it was at before the acute onset of his condition.

What to Do

Everything we've discussed so far in this chapter assumes a spousal sexual relationship—that is, one of long standing, whether or not you are married. If, in fact, you have a new relationship, that changes matters entirely. The primordial cardiology joke is for the doctor to say, when asked by a male patient if it's OK to have sex yet, "Sure, go ahead. But make sure it's with your wife. I don't want you to get too excited." The more modern version comes from a rehab expert who was consulted by a general practitioner about his recovering heart patient. The man's exercise level was up to 3.5 METs and the chart listed, among permitted activities at that level, "Sex (Marital)."* But, said the GP, how about extramarital sex? "No," said the rehab expert. "That's in the category of competitive sports—and that's 10 METs!"

However infuriating wives may find the joke, it has a valid point. We all became habituated to *any* activity. We find anything new more stressful, which certainly goes for sexual partners. Stress tapers off with the same partner and remains at a fairly low level, stabilized throughout the relationship. Not that pleasure is necessarily lessened (that's a compound of many factors), just the novelty, which produces the level of stress contraindicated for a recovering heart and body.

This points the way to what both of you can do about early post-coronary sex.

The doctor's permission to resume sex is predicated on a long-standing relationship because doctors recognize its low stress level. A

---

* Actually, METs measurements with regard to sex are a little complicated. As Dr. William Dafoe points out, with the demands of certain, sudden activities—including sex—the heart's oxygen requirement may be sharply high even though the body's overall METs requirement remains modest. Check with *your* doctor or rehab expert about *your* case.

decade ago, a doctor might say it was all right to resume sex when the patient could walk around the block 12 times or some such, though only twice around the block equalled the known stress of sex with a longstanding partner. The other 10 constituted a safety factor. Nowadays, doctors know that the heart can take—indeed *needs*—much more activity than they had imagined a decade ago. But they still figure in that safety factor. When a doctor, knowing you and the patient have enjoyed a longstanding relationship, says it's all right to resume sex, the doctor is not taking any chances and neither are you. The doctor *knows* the patient's heart will positively thrive on the amount of stress represented by sex, knows it empirically. That's because of those stress tests that may have begun even in the first few days of hospital stay, with the patient chugging away on a stationary bicycle or treadmill while hooked up to a monitor. Their purpose is to determine precisely the heart's reaction to measured levels of activity.

So the doctor has already *seen* the patient's heart easily accommodate much more stress than the amount generated by sexual activity. Sexual activity, that is, with a partner of long standing. That's the kicker: the stress level of sexual *novelty* necessarily remains an unknown for each couple, and at first the doctor will forbid it. Doctors do not cavalierly take chances with their patients' health—and it's easy enough to say "no" to someone else's sex life! If you're newlyweds,* or just a new item, most sex has to wait a while. Conversely, if yours is a longstanding relationship, there simply is no danger within whatever limits the doctor specifies.

What you can do is make sure the doctor thoroughly ventilates the subject with both you and the patient present. Don't be content with anything like "You can start sex in a week" or even "You can start right now"; insist that the doctor explain the reasoning behind that permission and the reasoning for any restrictions. That should dissipate any apprehension on everyone's part.

We use the word "insist" on purpose. Dr. Goldburgh is right about today's "more relaxed acceptance" of sexuality; but for some, "more relaxed" still equals "uptight." Even if you feel comfortable, the doctor may not, and if you sense reticence to discuss sex (or discover it in yourself) you must swallow hard and *insist*. The subject and its consequences are too important to be smothered by prudery or priggishness. Which would you rather endure: at worst, 10 minutes of embarrassment or months of anxiety?

---

* Significantly, newlywed sex creates more stress than premarital sex for the same couple. Suddenly, they have more to prove to themselves and each other.

You want to know exactly when you can do what. As Dr. Koller put it,

> The typical position, you know, is "male-on-top." But there are lots of others. For a patient who still has a lot of weight to lose, being on top would present a very difficult problem, because it is kind of a push-up that involves isometric exercise, and isometric exercise is dangerous for heart patients. But with female-on-top, unless he tries to lift both of them off the bed, there's not that much risk. Side-by-side is not bad, and rear entry is certainly one of the least strenuous positions for the male.
>
> Also there's the whole area of experimentation with foreplay and stimulation on both sides. None of that is even particularly stressful, certainly nothing like ejaculation or orgasm during intercourse.

Each couple is different because each heart condition is. Does the doctor suggest or prohibit any particular positions or activities for you? If so, why? and for how long? If full sexual activity is out for any length of time, how about the stimulation Dr. Koller mentioned? Is it all right to induce orgasm without intercourse through oral sex or masturbation? If not right away, when? You need specific, "hardcore" answers.

It's not inconceivable that you had some sexual problems long before any heart condition became an issue. If in fact they were heart-related even if you didn't realize it (as with angina pain, discussed above), they will now disappear. For others, if you made sexual adjustments and accommodations before, you will easily do so again. The message of this chapter is: *the heart condition need in no way interfere.*

CHAPTER 14

Divorce Cardiac-style

Attitude
Divorce, FINAL
Divorce, "Happy"
Divorce, Undone

Attitude

Maybe you and the patient have already separated; maybe you were about to be separated, or were discussing it. Then the heart condition came to crisis, and now you are not sure what to do. Call off the divorce? Postpone any further action? Go ahead? Let's weigh the probable consequences of each course.

Unless you enjoy martyrdom, deciding unilaterally now to call off proceedings makes little sense. As we'll see in "Divorce, Undone," below, conditions that led to the split may have changed; a divorce may no longer be necessary. But it's certainly too early to tell, and there's no reason to commit yourself to promises you may later either regret or have to break.

Then should you postpone any further action? For your own sense of self-worth and non-guilt, that intuitively seems the answer. One woman, on the edge of divorce when her husband suffered a heart attack, told us why she had put it off:

> What kind of woman does something like that? Walking out on a sick man! Why, they'd throw rocks at you!

She would have cast the first. If you walk away now, you give yourself maximum opportunity to feel guilty. Either the patient never fully recovers (worse, dies); then how will you feel about the effect your leaving might have had and what will your answer to that question do to you? Or the patient recovers; then how will you feel about yourself for not having helped? And what kind of shape will those feelings leave you in for someone else who may someday need you?

Postponement seems to make sense, but is by no means an automatic decision. The trouble is that unless you give almost constant thought to your position, the relationship with your spouse will probably degenerate into the patterns of word and deed that led to your wanting a divorce in the first place. Your feelings toward your spouse do not figure to be generous and kindly, yet that's often what's needed in *happy* marriages, given some of the aberrations in personality and behavior we've discussed throughout the book. Now, outrageous behavior that is merely the characteristic aftermath of a heart condition may seem just another page in the same old story. Without thinking, you may react to it the same old way, giving tit-for-tat what you get.

But this is a new story, with new complications. If the atmosphere of recovery is envenomed by bitter quarrels and by choking, heart-pounding rages—well, the heart can take a lot more than cardiologists thought a decade ago, but who knows?

Then, if being part of recovery holds its dangers, should you go ahead with the divorce? We've already explained the more probable dangers of that option. Although that seems to leave you with *no* choices, the solution lies in postponement with an *unshakable* commitment to a useful, pragmatic attitude.

All the information in this book applies to you as much as to someone happily married. You face the same problems, and must do the same things to help speed recovery. The difference is why you do them and in what spirit. Those with happy marriages want to keep them; they do what must be done, putting up with the hardships and unpleasantnesses willingly and with love. You have a miserable marriage; you can hope to salvage from it only a "happy" divorce, one leaving you emotionally free to start again. That makes your job harder. Much will happen that is hard enough to put up with even for the sake of a happy marriage. For you, unpleasantness takes place against the background of an already failed marriage. You will be unsustained by the motives of love. Still, if you can cope with the problems, you will walk away from the marriage with a free mind, an easy conscience, and clear emotions. Your attitude must be: This, too, shall pass, and I'll put up with it all because (forgetting any residual affection or pity for the patient) doing so is the wisest course for my own future emotional well-being. That is divorce, cardiac-style.

Actually, it's the third kind. In all, there are five. We examine the first two in "Divorce, FINAL," the third in "Divorce, 'Happy,'" and the last two (a pleasant surprise) in "Divorce, Undone."

Good luck with whatever you choose.

Divorce, FINAL

This is really a holdover from *Survive,* when cardiologists thought a damaged heart could take a lot less of the pounding stress engendered by violent emotions than they now know to be true. But the change just makes these two kinds of truly *final* divorce less easy or less likely than we first imagined. The point remains valid.

You will find a chilling picture of the first kind in Eugene O'Neill's play *Mourning Becomes Electra.* In the Greek myth, when Agamemnon comes home from the Trojan War, his wife and her lover kill him. O'Neill set the story in New England at the end of the Civil War. General Ezra Mannon, in his fifties, married to a younger woman who loathes him and loves a sea captain, has a "weak heart." First, Christine tries "loving" Ezra to death. As any rehab expert (or reader of our chapters 11 and 13) could tell her, that method was almost bound to fail—save, perhaps, from the effect of surprised shock: Ezra did not get much loving before he went off to war. Undaunted, Christine next tries something more sensible. She throws her infidelity in Ezra's face, with infuriating details. As she hopes, his rage triggers another attack, her chance to switch poison for his usual medicine.

Actually, poison may be superfluous, even given what we know today about the heart's resilience. With all a spouse's opportunities, especially considering the strain of estrangement, he or she might be able to generate enough tension, turmoil, and chaos to see the ailing spouse keel over within a month of leaving the CCU. That is the first kind of divorce, cardiac-style, the truly final decree, without any tiresome waiting, lawyers to pay, property to divide, custody fights. The survivor gets everything, even sympathy!

The second kind is the same, minus malign intentions. Instead of design, it sees the couple gravitate to a replay of all the wrangling and acerbity that inspired thoughts of divorce in the first place. The progression is easy. The stresses of forced intimacy during illness and convalescence aggravate the natural animus of a couple who were, anyway, about to split; words lead to words, and soon the words are shouted, hearts pounding.

True, this second kind of divorce, cardiac-style, has even less likelihood of a literally fatal outcome than does the first; you don't *mean* to fight and you probably don't press the attack when the results becomes plain. But it surely spells the death of the marriage and of your hopes of walking away with a clear conscience because you've helped recovery. Besides, if your very presence promotes such dangerous discord, even unintentionally, you're both better off rid of each other immediately.

Divorce, "Happy"

The basic conditions for, attitude about, and reasoning behind this kind of divorce, cardiac-style, are outlined above in "Attitude."

You simply put off any further action on the separation or divorce until your spouse is recovered. In this time of extreme need, you "stand by" the person you once thought enough of to marry, not because you necessarily feel that the person deserves it, but because you deserve a future free of guilt. For how long must you "stand by"? Until you know in *your* heart that the patient's heart is well enough for you to go off feeling good about what you have done.

There is no question of fooling your spouse about a change in your relationship. If you were separated, there is no need to pretend that everything is fine now and that you are coming back for good. If you were only discussing separation, ignore the discussions; if asked, say that it is something you both must put aside for now: recovery is important to both of you; your own immediate concern is helping it happen. If you were simply planning separation, forget it for now.

Mr. and Mrs. P had separated not much before symptoms of Mr. P's cardiomyopathy began to incapacitate him. She had asked him to leave, saying she did not really love him anymore and was, in fact, involved with someone else. When they had been apart for about a year, though not yet divorced, he received a transplant. They moved back together again when he came out of the hospital, and he said sometime later that during the recovery period,

> . . . for the first three months neither of us was working; we did something every day together. And it's strange: you seem to put everything else aside after an event like this. Nothing else matters, just the surgery and recovering. We didn't worry about anything; everything was wonderful. I was alive, and we didn't even think about the marriage.
>
> Then, after we got back to the routine of working, both with full time jobs, the attitude went back, and she started back on this business of "nothing's changed, and I want to start counseling again." And I said, "Cut it out right now. Whether God gives me two years or he gives me twenty, I'm not going to stay in a relationship like this."

Now the split was final.

Of course we're getting only the patient's point of view. But, consciously or not, Mrs. P got herself a "happy" divorce, cardiac-style.

Divorce, Undone

If you're going to have the fourth kind—a "divorce" not from the person but from the conditions that caused behaviors that made you want a divorce—you've actually already had it. It happened when doctors diagnosed and treated the heart condition.

Mrs. V, for instance, over a period of two years had watched her husband change into a bitter, narrow, miserably unhappy man. There was no explaining it, but her marriage seemed to be crumbling. Nothing she did seemed to matter. Nothing she suggested—counseling, therapy, changes of job or neighborhood or state—nothing was "worth trying," because "nothing could possibly make a difference," according to her increasingly strange, and estranged, husband. Then, one night, she got a phone call:

> I heard "hospital" and I thought, "It's an accident." The way he'd been,
> I hated to have him drive. I was sure he was going to kill himself.
>   When the intern said "heart attack," it was—well, almost a relief.
> I suddenly knew that's why he'd been like that!

As the coronary artery gets narrower, letting through increasingly less blood, the heart operates under increasing strain, pumps with decreasing efficiency. As the body gets less blood, the victim experiences a generally rotten feeling almost guaranteed to taint appreciation of everything, including you and your marriage. One of the symptoms of actual heart attack is a general, nonspecific "feeling of doom"; that feeling may have been building for years and may have been the cause of the disaffection between you.

If so, it may be past. Surgery or other therapy restored blood flow, relieved the symptoms. You may already have had your fourth kind of divorce, cardiac-style. You will have to wait a while to be sure; as you've seen, some of the stresses of recovery can result in behavior indistinguishable from whatever made you want a divorce. It is worth the wait!

The fifth kind is even more common, but more problematical since it is not at all automatic; it also takes longer.

Why was your marriage breaking up? If from a general, growing, freeform dislike, or total lack of mutual interest and respect— "incompatibility" in its real and personal, as opposed to merely legal, sense—then no, chances are your marriage cannot be saved, and most likely should not be. Divorce is the only remedy for true indifference. But if particular qualities (or lack of them), specific acts (or constant omissions) were making the marriage impossible, a chance remains.

Can you give the problem a single definitive name? Overambition? Laziness? Irresponsibility? Those are some of the usual problems. Even more usual is a basic immaturity, a childish attitude toward that great adult compromise called marriage. It can show up in surprising ways, such as chronic infidelity: not the kind that involves running off with someone, which at least signifies an adult willingness to make a choice, but "cheating" and "sneaking around," the sexual equivalent of the child's wanting to have a cake and eat it, too. Perhaps the most common problem is what's become known as "type A behavior": careerists so driven (and driving), so determined to "give their families *everything*" that what they really give them are neuroses, insecurity, an absentee parent and spouse, finally, a visit to the Coronary Care Unit.

If your marriage was being destroyed by any such problems, you may find that the heart condition has "divorced" the problems from personality or lifestyle—with luck, both. The intimations of mortality that accompany a heart condition very often impel patients to their first true self-assessment. The results can be startling and gratifying for both partners.

We've already met Mr. and Mrs. O (see chapter 9). Their marriage had been degenerating quite a while before doctors diagnosed his heart condition and performed bypass surgery. After about a year that saw Mr. O's almost total breakdown of personality, Mrs. O left him. We've heard some of what she has to say on the various aspects of the problem before, but her words bear repeating now because they reward pondering in this new light. When asked about her husband's change, she says:

> Because we had been separated, and for a year hadn't even seen each other, it came suddenly to me. He, of course, had been going through a tremendous upheaval. All I knew was that we slowly started seeing each other again, and I began to be aware that he was a different person altogether, different, even, from what he had been prior to the change. He had become very, very introspective and gentle. He had absolutely willed himself to stop being a high-pressure person.
>
> He had all the characteristics, you know, of a person who is a candidate for a heart attack. He isn't now.

Recalling the process, Mrs. O says,

> He did a lot of soul-searching. He took an honest look at himself and said, "I don't like what I see, and I'm going to change." It was hard for him to do because he had always had a volatile personality. He was always at the point of exploding, and frequently did. He just willed himself to get rid of that; it doesn't exist anymore.

What was the result of the introspection and willpower at least indirectly flowing from Mr. O's heart condition? And did it last? Mrs. O continues:

> He's a completely different person now. He's mellowed now; he's just a normal person now.

It's been over five years, and they are together, quite content. Of course they have problems, but only the normal problems of living. This is the kind of divorce, cardiac-style, every estranged cardiac couple might wish for.

CHAPTER 15

This Is Your Lives

(NOTE: Sybil Straker had successful heart surgery after years of struggling with defective valves. Her husband, who spoke with us four years after the surgery, is a psychiatrist.)

> Both of us know that we live until we die and it's the same process for everybody. We both feel blessed that we've lived to this age—we're both over 70 now—and we're very grateful for anything we have now.
>
> I don't mean that we're aware of that all the time; but it colors the way we react to our own ultimate mortality. The important thing is not if we die or don't die, but rather the quality of our life.
>
> —Dr. Manuel Straker

Attitude, Basic

We want to tell you a joke.

Two sparrows sat on a fence. Being especially dim sparrows, they never moved from that fence. The summer sun beat down on them; they choked in the dust, panted with thirst, ached with sunburn. In winter they shivered with cold, shook with chills, their feathers drooping and soggy in the snow and rain. Still they sat.

This went on for years. Finally one sparrow turned to the other and croaked hoarsely, "This sure is a rotten way to live, isn't it?"

The second sparrow's brow furrowed in thought. Then he turned to his companion and asked, "Compared with what?"

Aside from the few exceptions we've noted, anyone with a heart condition has that condition "for life," making the necessary mental and physical adjustments. It follows that the person's family becomes in some measure a "heart family," also for life, to greater or lesser degree participating in the same adjustments.

A rotten way to live?

Compared with what? The way you were living before? Something about that, or a combination of somethings, gave someone you love a heart condition and has been giving you a fair number of problems ever since. That's good? Whatever kind of life you live from now on cannot give you a much worse result. Certainly it will have to be different, but why should you assume it's bad? You haven't tried it yet.

The question is, *how* will the new life differ?

Start with the difference in your own life. A woman we know developed a severe case of diabetes in her late thirties. She had always been highly active, had five children and a large house to run; she also had a master's degree in city planning—acquired after the diabetes, when she found herself getting a little bored—and a part-time job as special admissions officer at a nearby university. We asked her whether diabetes had made much of a difference in how she lives. After pondering, she said, "Well . . . now I take insulin."

Exactly. She takes insulin. And she does not take certain other things: cake, candy, anything with a discernible sugar content. That may suggest that she does not take dessert; it depends on whether or not she has taken the time to plan ahead and the trouble to make an allowed dessert for herself. Before going on a trip, or being away from home all day, she must plan to have a supply of food with her and a supply of insulin and syringes. It is no big deal, if indeed she does plan.

Now *you* take thought about certain things. You plan. You learn. Sometimes you scheme. As one woman put it, "I learned to be a little crafty." Another woman, wife of a transplant patient, cheerfully admits almost two years after the operation,

> I find myself turning down—he doesn't know this [LAUGHS]—some invitations out for breakfast with a group from our church because I know where they're going to eat is a smorgasbord, all the goodies you're not supposed to eat.
>
> I find myself thinking, "No, we better not do it," because I know what temptation is, and best thing is to stay away from it in a case like that.

After a while the taking thought and planning become instinctive; equally so, as time passes you have less and less of it to do because everyone involved fairly quickly falls into the comfortable role of awareness as part of a Heart Family.

At that point, "problems" are the normal vagaries of living.

A rotten way to live? For whom? And what aspect of it?

Cooking? Eating? Recall the woman who said how much fun it was "fooling them all" with her cardiac cuisine, and the children who became, if anything, a little *too* fanatic about eating right, hectoring their poor father about every wrong bite; remember the delight of the family in which they *all* shed unwanted pounds.

Is exercise a burden? For whom? Recall that Polly Brown's favorite time of day is still twilight because it evokes memories of her delicious, quiet-time walks (i.e., prescribed exercise) with her heart-patient father.

Are you going to pine for the hectic qualities of living and self-generated stress that now must be curbed? A personal note. JoAnn still recalls the thrill of pride, several years after her husband's heart attack, when the phone rang at 2 a.m. and a distraught client wailed that his factory had just burned down. Forrest calmed the man, pointed out that neither of them could do anything useful at that hour, so they should both get a good night's rest and they'd examine the financial picture in the morning. Before the heart attack Forrest would surely have dashed down to the scene and stood about with the client, indeed accomplishing nothing but the attainment of a high stress level and a sleepless night.

A rotten way to live? No. Only a different way. And the difference is that, with the right attitude, the entire family lives a life that, just on the record of what havoc your pre-heart-condition life wreaked, makes much more sense and must contribute to an overall sense of greater satisfaction for every one of you.

Attitude, Changed

There is a "cardiac personality." Exceptions abound; but predominant among those who develop heart conditions are the more driving, tense, and compulsive. The cardiac experience goes a long way toward helping such people change. At a group meeting of cardiac couples, this exchange took place:

Mr. U: No one has assurance you're going to live on and on. You just live your life as best you can.

Mrs. S: Do you think the heart attack has taken the fun out of it, out of life?

Mr. U: Well, I don't know. I do think you take life a little more seriously. You think about it a little more.

Mr. C: I think it changes people's outlook. And this is where, eventually, you have people coming to settle down and realize what things really are.

I mean they get a grip on themselves and start saying, "Well, this is reality; this is the way things really are. And *this* is important—living happy." Whereas all those material things and power and being a big shot don't do it for you anymore.

You grow up a lot, without gray hairs.

So the answer to maturity is . . . go have a heart attack!

It's not just the patient; family members report the same kinds of changes. The wife of one patient told us,

It changes your personality. It changes you. I think it's made me much more tolerant, and certainly able to empathize with people more.

You will be much less uptight about everything. You will find that you have outgrown many of what had before seemed insurmountable problems. In large measure, that's what your lives as a Heart Family come down to: living lives that often make for more profound happiness and that make more sense to you. The circumstances and necessary adjustments of a heart condition forcibly strip away assumptions about how you "had" to live and what it takes to make you happy. Better still, a heart condition usually teaches its psychologic lessons without inflicting such physical damage as to render the knowledge useless.* Treatment is *not* curative, as we've often repeated; but no physical fact about a heart condition, adequately palliated with treatment, stands in the way of your constructing a life better than you enjoyed before. And that includes the threat of future complications or recurrences.

The husband of one woman suffered a number of heart attacks and finally died, 14 years after the first one. But until then, says the woman,

My husband said that the . . . years during the time he had his coronary condition were the happiest years of his life. . . . He was a very content man—he had an interesting, stimulating, and satisfying life.

Another woman, asked if there is any marked difference in quality of life between her first marriage and her second to a transplant recipient, says,

I didn't find that there is that much difference. Jim was always so active and a go-getter at anything he did. It crosses your mind he might have a heart attack again, but it's not something you sit around and dwell on.

---

* Like the circus performer who insisted on walking the high wire without a net, now lying in bed, totally paralyzed after a fall, saying, "Well it certainly was a lesson to me."

A changed attitude does it. Mr. K, a hard-charging lawyer, traveled a lot on both business and pleasure. His wife usually joined him on trips, and while she enjoyed them, she realized that they represented more to him: travel for him, says Mrs. K, was "really a passion." Indeed, she says, "our *life* had almost been the trips; I mean we could almost count the years as to where we were. We could think of 1972—oh, Turkey!"

His hectic practice ended with a heart attack and bypass surgery. The travel* would have to end for a period, too. The two of them took time to assess their lives. On reflection it made no sense to live only for the high spots, the trips. "We decided," says Mrs. K, "that *every day* had to be good. It meant putting ourselves where we could feel and be aware of changes of season and so forth. The day-to-day became very important." It was a big move. At an age when many couples move to apartments, they moved to a large property in a new community, what Mrs. K calls, "a bigger piece of grass to cut." And even that required an attitude change: a turning away from compulsive, perfectionist behavior and a new realization, says Mrs. K, "that if the grass isn't cut one week, it's not going to kill us." It was a huge change for them both. And, says Mrs. K, "The illness had a lot to do with the need for change."

Everyone in your family will lead many different lives, with many different interests, as a result of your patient's heart condition and the changes it brings to family life. The important thing is to stay open to change, to *try* things. You all will be amazed at how much you like.

Back to Work

Everything important about this was said by two people, a doctor and a patient. It applies equally to men and women, depending on how important their careers were to them. Dr. Hillel Laks, a cardiac surgeon, says:

> Unfortunately, when one looks at the record of bypass surgery, it's disappointing in that a large number of patients, who physically and medically are capable of working, do not go back to work, many of them for psychological and insurance and other reasons.
>
> But I think that without occupational rehabilitation, the surgery has not been completely successful. And the family should try to get patients back to work, either in their previous work or a new occupation.

---

* But only, as she puts it, "ceaseless" travel, not travel altogether; see "Travel," below.

Even patients who did heavy physical work, such as construction workers, certainly could be fully employed in another field.

Sometimes patients avoid going back because they and their families feel their jobs contributed to stress in the past. But there is no good evidence that occupational stress is necessarily bad for patients. It depends on how it's handled and what type of stress it is. Rehabilitation education in better coping with stress is useful. Some patients may have more stress being restless and unoccupied and depressed at home than if they had an occupation.

Mr. W worked 28 years for a large company as an electronics technician before his cardiomyopathy got so bad he had to quit. Eighteen months after a transplant, at age 58, he contemplated returning to work until retirement age. He says:

> A lot of people say, "Why would you want to go back to work?" I say, [LAUGHING] "When you lay around four, five, six years and *can't* do anything when you feel like doing something, you jump at the chance to go back. You don't just want to lay there and die. You've got to keep active."

All the above is true *even if the patient for any valid reason cannot return to work* (see "Cardiac Cripple," below).

Cardiac Cripples, NOT Making

Three months after his bypass surgery, Mr. B was back playing tennis. "The doctor," says Mrs. B, "wanted Don to talk with other heart patients. He said, 'I wish more of my patients had half of your enthusiasm for recovery; you'd be surprised at how many people debilitate themselves: they turn themselves into cardiac cripples.'"

Many, like Mr. B, are determined from the first to get on with their lives. Too many others, aware that they can never be "cured," make the mistake of thinking that the symptoms must also linger on, uncurable. They indeed become cardiac cripples, unwilling to do much of anything, afraid to *live* for fear it might kill them. Sad, if understandable. As clinical coordinator Albert McClure points out,

> A lot of people who leave the hospital after a heart attack or heart surgery no longer see themselves as immortal, but as a cardiac cripple or invalid. And they don't do anything from that point forward for the rest of their life.
>
> They live without any idea or feeling that they control their destiny in any way.

Amazingly, the same applies even for transplant patients snatched back from the brink of the grave. "A lot of these patients were down to days, weeks, months at most," says Bernie Robbins, a rehab specialist. "They've been given a new lease on life. But a lot of them are just sitting and watching the rain fall."

It's bad enough that many patients share a propensity toward becoming cardiac cripples; it's worse when their families unwittingly propel them into that tragic state. "Patients walk a very fine line between full recovery and becoming invalids," says Carole Landers, another rehab specialist. "It doesn't take much. And sometimes families, spouses especially, are overprotective." Professionals are particularly annoyed when they see patients struggling to make a full comeback, only to be hampered by well-meaning but dead-wrong families. As Albert McClure says,

> A lot of patients want to know when they can do certain things: golf, driving, gardening, mowing the yard.
>
> The family often becomes overprotective at that point. They're saying, "Well, he wants to go do so-and-so, but I know he can't do that for so many weeks."
>
> And I say, "No, that's not true! he *can* do that!"
>
> They almost want to make an invalid of the patient—out of love, to be *sure* he's all right. But that's the worst thing you could do, to have someone recuperating from surgery or a heart attack and not allow them to do anything.

It's not simply a question, either, of what the family says; what they do, how they treat the patient, speaks volumes. If you treat someone like an invalid it often becomes what's called a "self-fulfilling prophecy." The most common example of this phenomenon occurs in sports, where you "psych" your opponents, convincing them they are so overmatched, they might as well not bother trying. Once they believe it and start telling themselves the same thing—in effect, prophesying their own defeat—they do not play to win. Not trying, they do lose, and the prophecy has fulfilled itself.

Of course, you can "psych" yourself, as well, positively ("I can't lose") and negatively ("I can't win"). Patients who prophesy their own infirmity make themselves cardiac cripples. People who treat them like invalids, by word or deed, prophesy the same thing, often with the same result.

What *is* treating people like invalids? Roughly, everything you do or say that proceeds from the assumption that people are invalids, continuing to do things for them long after they should be doing for themselves. One man we spoke to years ago recognized the danger and expressed it exactly:

> Listen—if I didn't get up and going, I could just sit around and let my darling wife be my darling wife and wait on me hand and foot. And she would gladly to it! Nothing's too much for her!

But if I let her, okay, I might as well crawl into a wheelchair and have a sign on my neck, "I am an invalid."

What, instead, do professionals want you to do? "I want," says clinical coordinator Kim Wimsatt,

the family to support the patient in recovering fully, not to make the patient a cardiac cripple. I want them to *know* the patient's getting well.

If we're talking about, say, angioplasty, I want the family to realize that when they get home not to walk on egg shells, and not to worry at every twinge that they have to rush the patient to the emergency room.

I want them to feel confident and comfortable with this situation, and feel that the more they know about it, the more the family and the patient are going to be able to live a normal life.

Is that too much to ask? During the years when doctors were insisting that Mrs. Straker's valve condition was inoperable, when she just had to live with it, she and her husband determined that she would indeed *live*. "When she was doing a little better," says Dr. Straker,

we tried to carry on as normally as possible. I didn't want to complete the process of "invaliding" her by having her under supervision 24 hours a day. She was encouraged to do, and, in fact, insisted on doing, all that she could on her own. That included shopping, driving the car, visiting, doing whatever housework she could, cooking, baking, maintaining our normal social life, entertaining, and so on.

When they discovered that her condition was indeed operable, guess what kind of recovery Mrs. Straker made.

So far we've been negative: DON'T make cardiac cripples of people you love. What positive steps can the family take to help ensure the speediest, most complete, most long-range recovery possible?

As usual, it starts with a correct attitude, and what you say. Never allow the patient, unchallenged, to express by word or deed the defeatism and self-pity of the cardiac cripple. One transplant patient credits her mother with a large part of her fine recovery. "When I had to be on crutches the first few weeks because of the prednisone,"* says Mrs. F, "she'd say, 'Big deal! Maybe tomorrow you won't be on crutches; but you should be thrilled you're alive to *be* on crutches.'"

The wife of another transplant patient says that, from time to time, when she sees her husband moping, or seriously slacking off from ongoing rehabilitative exercise or sensible eating, she puts it to him bluntly:

---

* Anti-rejection medicine with sometimes fearsome side effects.

"That's enough. A lot of people have serious illnesses." I have to remind him, "Some people have cancer, and they're dying."

"OK, you had a heart attack. Now you have a new heart; you're on your two feet; you have a brain; you can work; what's your problem?"

"Or, sometimes," she says, "I'll use diversion: I'll say, 'Why don't you call up Bob and go play golf?' Or, 'Let's go see Whitney.'" [Their granddaughter.]

The distinction is important and depends on circumstances. "You have to deal with people differently at different times, depending on circumstances and how they feel," says the same woman:

I can tell by the way he reacts, I can't be tough on him; that's when I have to use diversion.

Then, other times when I think he's just being a baby, when something hasn't gone his way and he's down and won't do anything, I'll just say, "Look! Are you gonna live this way? This is fun? You call this fun?"

You have to handle the situation as you go.

The issue of medication is a good place to start. Of all a patient's activities, this is the most personal, the one for which each should most be willing to take responsibility. A wife says,

I always tell the wives at the hospital support group meetings: "When you go home and get back into your routine, don't ever go get his medicine for him unless he's sick or he really feels bad."

Start with the medicine!

Watch and make sure he takes it, at first, but don't you go get it.

I think there were times when Harry waited until the last minute to see if I would go do it. Sometimes they test you, how much you care for them. Just to see if I care enough, he's not going to get his medicine. And I've let him wait 15, 20 minutes.

Of course, if he's asleep, or I know he feels bad, or he's forgotten, I say, "Harry, it's time for your medicine." But if I know he's just testing me, we have a little testing time.

This game of "medication chicken" has a point. *Truly* caring means encouraging the person to get well, not to contribute to infirmity. Start there and build.

Children

For those who already have children, and have all of them they ever intended to have, see chapter 12. But with the steadily lowering age for the onset of heart conditions, more families face the question of whether to have children (or more children) *now.*

Plainly, there is no single answer; it's too personal a question, with too many variables depending on personality and circumstance. But it may help to explore some possible ways of thinking about the problem.

First, we understand from doctors that, absent any unusual circumstances (you obviously have to consult your own doctor), a heart condition does not automatically bar pregnancy, even if the patient is the female. For a male patient, his wife's pregnancy is positively therapeutic, the best possible antidote to any lingering crises of masculinity brought on by the condition. Furthermore, for both, helping and supporting each other through the pregnancy and delivery constitutes for patients of either sex a bracing change from self-worries and self-doubts, and from the typical self-absorption of cardiac patients.

Obviously, this movement away from self-absorption grows geometrically with the normal demands of child rearing.

Against that, you should weigh at least two counterarguments. They were summed up for us years ago at a meeting of heart patients when a man in his middle twenties said that, although at the time of his heart attack he and his wife had decided to start a family, now she hesitated. Suppose he had another attack, this one fatal? She would end up raising the children alone. Besides, was it right to raise children when their father *might* have to restrict his activities, if not immediately, then perhaps in the future, and may not be the sort of father he wants to be?

Those are not trivial concerns. The wife of a different patient addressed the same doubts and came to a different conclusion:

> The hardest decision was determining whether or not we should have another child. I always felt I didn't want to take on any huge commitments that will create a lot of pressure for him.
>
> But we decided, Yes. We did not want to give up that delight.
>
> And I'm glad we did.

Frankly, we are a little ill at ease discussing this problem because we were both so lucky, having had all the children we had planned prior to our husbands' heart conditions. What's more, the children were old enough, and our husbands made rapid enough recoveries, so even in those days there was little question of their not participating in the children's lives. It's easy enough for us to talk. But we feel that "not giving up that delight" says it all. Just be aware that it should be a considered, and discussed, decision.

Hovering

The word conjures a picture of a hand-wringing spouse lurking just outside the door, waiting for any sound that might suggest the patient needs anything from a glass of water to an ambulance. The atmosphere is heavy with the apprehensive prophecy of chronic invalidism. In the early stages, it could destroy recovery. Later, it could destroy a marriage or a family.

Only two things need to be said about hovering for the entire family forever.

1. Don't.
2. See "Cardiac Cripples," above.

Pleasures, Assorted, Continuing

If yours is like most of the Heart Families we know, you will find that the pleasures of your life are not merely now-and-then compensations for the problems, but the dominant factor. The following "statistics" are entirely unreliable mathematically; we're just guessing as to the numbers. But we are convinced the spirit behind them is an accurate reflection of reality.

Ninety percent of the spouses we have talked with over the years feel their lives are better now, their marriages stronger now, and that they, the patient, and their families are better adjusted and happier now than before the onset of the condition.

Under 5% felt their lives, marriages, etc. were not satisfactory. And of those, most felt their "etc." were no great shakes before, either.

The remainder felt that while the aftermath of the heart condition had not made anything noticeably better for them, the patient was somewhat better off.

One wife told us:

We found out, for the first time in our lives—as individuals, and together in our married life—we found out what was important and what wasn't important. Before, we took everything for granted. Each other, too. And the children. All at once, you can't take anything for granted. So you stop and think.

We do much better now. Every way!

Finding pleasure in what most take for granted is especially common for those who have themselves suffered long periods of debilitation because of their condition before treatment, and for those family members who suffered along with them. One woman, who fought through 16 years of deterioration before she received a transplant, now works in her family business only three days a week—though she loves the work!—so she can spend more time with children. Not her own; she missed that pleasure: a nanny brought them up because she was usually too weak to care for them, even to lift them. Now, often as possible, she takes care of her younger brother's children. Before, she says, everything was bland; now she appreciates her house, her car, her life. "Now," she says,

> I *participate!* I never made menu plans; the cook had to do it. Now I go to the market. I fill my own car with gas!
> We have a cook and a housekeeper, but I clean this house because I *can* now. And Conrad says, "What are you doing?" and I say, "I'm having so much fun! I couldn't do it before. I don't want to fire anybody, but . . . I wash my car!"

And what does Conrad say? He notes how much closer his wife and their daughter are now. And he sums up with, "This is fabulous, the best years of our marriage." *And this couple went through, if anything, more than the usual number of recovery and rehab problems.*

What accounts for the life of pleasures that you can expect after a reasonable family adjustment to a heart condition? A good deal of it is the new openness that results from the characteristic change of attitude we examined in that entry, above. A willingness to look at life and savor what you find truly worthwhile. The wife told us this years ago:

> The year after his heart attack, we went to Europe. He finally decided he's going to do the whole thing, everything he always talked about. Now! At last! You know: "I'm going to do what I want to do and to hell with making a little more money just so I can pay bigger taxes!"
> I'm sure every woman tells you the same thing: that it changed her husband's attitude about everything. His whole approach to life.
> And I think it's so much healthier! If they only had that attitude before, maybe they wouldn't get the heart attacks in the first place. You only live once. You can only make so much money. And why, if you don't have time to enjoy it?
> Why should it take a heart attack to make a man see that?

Surely she didn't mean that somehow a heart attack or other heart condition was some kind of *good.* We wouldn't, we told her, want to see anybody have a heart problem, to risk death, just to find out how to live. "Well, I would!" she said,

> if *that's* what it takes. Because the other isn't living.
> I've seen it in so many men with heart attacks! They don't start to live until they nearly die.
> I don't mean just the trip, for my husband. Everything! How he lives and enjoys it now; he even enjoys his work more now.

Credit the openness engendered by enforced change. Suddenly the whole family will find profound satisfaction in things they otherwise simply would never have tried: like Polly as a little girl on twilight walks with Daddy; like the high-powered lawyer whose only pleasure had been travel until he and his wife decided that *every day* had to be good.

Your own pleasures will be equally unexpected and gratifying.

Role Reversals and Reestablishment*

This becomes less crucial as the sexes grow to share more of the traditional "duties" of each—call it feminism or lib or what you will—because then the relinquishing and reassumption of various roles are burdened with less and less emotional baggage. For now, though, it can still be a problem.

Most common is role reversal between spouses, especially with a male patient. The less sharing the marriage has been, and the more serious the heart condition, requiring the patient to relinquish more, the more pronounced chances are for conflict. Of course this presents no problem if the newly empowered spouse doesn't care. During an unusually long, complex convalescence, Mrs. H found herself making arrangements, speaking out. "I've learned to talk," she says. "Jim did all the talking, planning, and all that, before. That's been a big change." She does not relish the change. "I want it to go back. I mean, I don't mind doing it, but I'd rather have him more in charge."

The reaction is more often like that of Mrs. A, who says, "He didn't like it very much, but I just said to him, 'You know, I got a taste of what it's like to have some of the power and I like it; it's been too long the other way.' We've been married 18 years, and there were times when he was intimidating and I wasn't liberated enough."

For those situations, clinical coordinator Bobbie Scallorn sketches the scenario for some:

> The longer patients have been sick, the more they've given up control of their lives. They've given up their jobs, handling the check book, giving advice to the family members, decision-making. And now they've got somebody telling them when to have an appointment, when to take their medicine.
>
> The family may start feeding on this new power they've taken over, and it can become a real dynamic problem.
>
> It's hard to regain control after you've given it up. It's hard for the wife who's now writing the check to say, "Here, I want you to do this, I don't want to do it"—especially if she's never had control, and now she's the important person in the family and even more if she feels she's doing a better job of it!

---

* This subject tends to be more important for men than for women, and for the older, rather than the younger generation; but it applies in some measure to all.

> Like with one of my transplant patients who's depressed. I feel if he could take back some of the authority, some of the things that supposedly a man controls, he would do better.

For the long run, it's vital that patients be able to reassert enough of their roles so that they feel comfortable with themselves. Polly Brown, discussing personality change, noted how men, especially, even while still in the hospital, will sometimes "pick a quarrel in order to take the upper hand again." Later on, if they haven't made an adjustment, the result can be the depression Scallorn speaks of, even getting serious enough to create another cardiac cripple. "I get calls," says Brown,

> from patients, or from their wives, saying, "Joe is just blue; I can't get him to do anything, I'm here with him all the time."
> And I say, "Well, wait just a minute! He needs to reestablish his independence; you can't hang over him all the time. You're not his mother, you're his wife."
> You need to reestablish that relationship.

What's the answer? Strangely enough it's not love so much as it is good will, respect, fairness, and a sense of self-interest that can evaluate the longer-range good. It may not be easy to encourage a return in *any* degree to what the family may now see as an intolerable former status quo. But everyone's best interests are plainly served by encouraging the patient to make the most complete recovery.

Must the family realignment realign "power"? Very well, you can reasonably work out the give and take necessary, even have "treaty" discussions. A wife can make it clear that she wants not to ursurp her husband's place, but simply to continue with more participation in family finances; a husband can make it clear to his patient wife that he has no intention of replacing her as mother, but the taste he's necessarily had of being closer to the children makes him want to continue to be a more participatory father; a child can claim the rights of adulthood already exercised during the crisis. It all simply needs that infusion of good will, plus the realization on all sides that you are, after all, a *family* searching for the best way that all of you can live.

Travel

As we mention above in "Attitude, Changed," the lawyer whose passion was travel had to cut back, but certainly did not have to eliminate travel. Virtually no one has to forego that pleasure just because of a heart condition. For one thing, medical standards throughout much of the world, today, are such that you can find more than adequate care in an emergency.

Here's a short list of suggestions to help you plan.

- Tuck a copy of the latest EKG in a travel bag, along with copies of all prescriptions (including for eyeglasses, of which it's a good idea, anyway, to take an extra pair), a small flashlight, and a spoon for mixing and measuring doses.

- Take extra medication along, each in a plastic bag, plus a list of medications and doses.

- If your doctor knows of reliable doctors and/or hospitals (especially those with coronary care units) where you're headed, take names, addresses, and phone numbers with you. Otherwise (maybe also), join one of the organizations described below.

- Make sure you carry with you the names and addresses of your home doctor and of relatives who know about your condition.

- If you harbor any allergies to any medications, make sure they're listed and easily found.

- Make sure you have luggage with wheels on the big pieces; porters are not universally available.

- Space your travel to leave yourself a day or two of rest between each leg; try to arrange for as few as possible early departures and late arrivals.

- If you have any eating restrictions, tote along emergency supplies—such as little cans of salt-free tuna, crackers, trail mix, packets of instant oatmeal.

- Call ahead to order any special airline meals—such as low-sodium or low-fat—you might need.

- Check with the American Heart Association for approved restaurants at your destinations.

A few minutes thought will provide you with a list of other precautions suited to your particular needs. None of the planning time is wasted. In the overwhelming likelihood that everything goes splendidly and there's no call for any of the precautions, your trip will anyway be more carefree, knowing you've covered the foreseeable.

One thing that is wise for anyone with a heart condition, and really essential to everyone's piece of mind when traveling, is membership in Medic Alert International. Members receive an engraved bracelet (or, if you choose, necklace) that alerts medical personnel to the patient's health problem, including allergies. For membership information, call the toll-free number: (800) 432–5378 (the last seven digits of which, you may notice, spell ID ALERT).

American Express offers card holders a service called Global Assist, a 24-hour hotline for medical (and legal) referrals around the world. (Several other credit card companies offer similar services.) If you're more than 100 miles away from home, the service can give you the names of doctors, hospitals, dentists, pharmacies, etc., in your area; if there's a language problem, they'll set up appointments. In addition, they'll relay emergency messages for you, send you hard-to-get medications, and will do a raft of other useful things, making this a very attractive travel package.

In addition, Global Assist lets you purchase very reasonable travel insurance called Travel Assistance International; this differs from most travel insurance in useful ways, providing not only trip cancellation reimbursement, but also overseas medical help, including the services of people who speak the local language if you need them; it also pays for medical treatment.

You qualify for Global Assist simply by being a member of American Express. For information, call toll-free (800) 554–2639 (the last four digits spell AMEX; you'll just have to remember the 554 on your own). You can purchase Travel Assistance International insurance by itself (it's a separate company). That phone number is (800) 821–2828, which doesn't spell anything, but is toll-free.

Finally, you might want to join IAMAT—International Association for Medical Assistance to Travellers—which offers a frequently updated worldwide list of centers (often hospitals, otherwise IAMAT offices) that will refer members to nearby approved doctors; "approved" means able to speak English, with professional qualifications reviewed to be sure they are up to IAMAT standards, and willing to treat members at remarkably reasonable set rates. IAMAT is nonprofit; membership and their directory are free. IAMAT depends on volunteers and donations. The address for information is 417 Center Street, Lewiston, NY 14092, the phone (716) 754–4883.

Have a nice trip, and don't forget to write!

Word, A Final

Although we admit she had a considerable point, we still disagree with the woman we quoted above in "Pleasures" who said that if it takes a heart condition to bring people to their senses about how they are living and how they should be living, then so be it, she'd wish them a heart condition. A permanent life-threatening condition seems a high price to pay even for the boon of sane living.

But in the case of you and your family there's no choice.

The heart condition is an irreversible, inescapable fact. Only one question remains: having unavoidably paid the price, will you seize the benefit?

Ernest Hemingway once defined life as "one damn thing after another." As we write this, a book by the late comedian Gilda Radner has appeared, an account of what turned out to be her fatal illness, called *It's Always Something.*

So it is; and indeed it is one something after another. But they are decidedly not all automatically damnable. Some are good, some bad. All *are* (except the fatal ones, of course) to some degree what you make of them.

The heart condition, by itself, is nothing. What you do about it, the adjustments you make, the lessons you learn—they are everything. No area in the conduct of your life depends more directly on your own actions and attitude. We don't mean the quality of your life in general; that still depends on all the factors that were operative before the heart condition, and that will continue to influence your existence. We mean the *difference* in your entire family's life as a result of the heart condition. That difference depends almost exclusively on what you and your family make of it.

Yes, it is a different life. But, depending on how you approach it, it can be a wonderful difference, a wonderful life. Yes, you do give up some things. But you find that for the most part they are things that brought you scant pleasure before. You give up a little to get a lot, including closer, richer relationships throughout your family born of your need to rally around and help one another.

Five years, ten years, twenty and more years from now, if someone asks you what kind of life you are leading as a Heart Family, you will wonder, "compared with what?" Because it will be hard for you to imagine that you could ever have led, or wanted to, any other kind.

And you are not alone.

Acknowledgments

First comes our deep gratitude to the many people who generously took the time and trouble to talk with us, and to share with you, through us, their wisdom, experience, and expertise. Without them, this book obviously would not have been possible.

Those who were coronary patients, or relatives (usually spouses) of patients, remain anonymous. We wanted to encourage the utmost candor about their experiences and emotions, and anonymity best assures that. The doctors, nurses, and other health care professionals who contributed so much to this book are listed, with their titles and professional affiliations, at the beginning of Notes.

We also relied on the help of some patients, spouses, and professionals who contributed to our first book, and whose help we acknowledged at greater length there. We repeat that thanks.

A host of people, some family, all dear friends, made our research much easier and infinitely more pleasant. A geographic listing gives you some idea of the range of encouragement, interview arrangements, and hospitality we received:

Boston: Hazel Cherney, John and Joy Pratt

Chicago: Michael Becker, Gertrude Grais, Elaine Kaplan and Joel Lee

Connecticut: Rob and Dale Rosen

Los Angeles: Selma Strock, Lois Marcum (La Quinta)

New Jersey: Max and Sadie Atkins, Jerry and Sylvia Atkins,

Jack and Bea Atkins, Verna Atkins, Emily and Bob Korb,
David and JaneEllen Gerstein, Mel and Gayle Gerstein,
Norma and Norman Nutman, Steven and Daryl Roth
  New York: Irving and Muriel Gerstein, Nick and Janet Wedge
(Ossining)
  Ottawa: Max and Helen Vechter
  Philadelphia: Burt and Shirley Wellenbach
  San Antonio: Lewis and Charlotte Lee
  Toronto: Marion Orenstein

We thank these people for their help and advice: Judith A.
Battaglia, Account Manager, Europ Assistance World Wide Services,
American Express; Denise M. Damron and Patrick Stone of Humana
Heart Institute; Herm Perlmutter, Community Programs Specialist,
American Heart Association; Harriet Roth, dietitian and author.

We thank Charles Phillips for sharing with us some interviews he
conducted at Vanderbilt University Hospital with transplant patients
for the book he wrote with Dr. William Frist. The book is *Transplant:
The Life and Death Struggle of a Heart Surgeon in the Frontier of
the New Medicine* (Morgan Entrekin/Atlantic Monthly Press, 1989).
Interviews conducted by Mr. Phillips are identified in Notes.

We had the inestimable benefit of medical advice and guidance
from a number of physicians: Drs. Len Davis, Richard N. Fine,
Mohammad Malek, Philip Marcus; and from research immunologist
Michael Cecka, Ph.D. All were most generous with their time and
patience in answering our questions, heading us in useful directions,
in many cases reading and critiquing all or part of the manuscript.
Any errors that have survived are due to our incomprehension, not
their care and caring.

We would like to express our special gratitude to Arthur Schoenberg's personal physicians: Drs. Kobashigawa, Kawata, and
Moriguchi.

We thank Lois Marcum for editing help.

Finally, we thank Robert J. Schoenberg for his help at every step
in the preparation of this book.

Notes and Sources

Where we cite the source of facts or quotations in the text, we do not further note them here. When the source is one of the professionals we interviewed for this book, we identify each with the person's last name. Their full names and professional affiliations are:

ALPERN, Harvey, M.D.; private practice, preventive cardiology, Century City; Clinical Chief, Cardiac Rehabilitation, Cedars-Sinai Medical Center, Los Angeles

BOWLBY, Mary; Dietitian; University of Ottawa Heart Institute Prevention and Rehabilitation Centre at the Ottawa Civic Hospital

BROWN, Polly, R.N.; Clinical Director; Humana Heart Institute International, Louisville

COHN, Lawrence H., M.D.; Chief of Cardiac Surgery; Brigham & Women's Hospital, Boston

CUPPER, Laura, R.N.; Vocational Rehabilitation Counselor; University of Ottawa Heart Institute Prevention and Rehabilitation Centre at the Ottawa Civic Hospital

DAFOE, William, M.D., F.R.C.P.(C); Director, Prevention and Rehabilitation Dept.; University of Ottawa Heart Institute Prevention and Rehabilitation Centre at the Ottawa Civic Hospital

DeVRIES, William C., M.D.; Cardiovascular Surgeon; Humana Hospital Audubon, Louisville

FRIST, William H., M.D.; Director, The Vanderbilt Transplant Center, Vanderbilt University Hospital, Nashville

GANZ, William, M.D.; private practice; Cedars-Sinai Medical Center, Los Angeles

GIBSON, Kim; Occupational Therapist; University of Ottawa Heart Institute Prevention and Rehabilitation Centre at the Ottawa Civic Hospital

GIRARDET, Roland E., M.D.; Staff Surgeon; Humana Heart Institute International, Louisville

GOLDBURGH, Warren, M.D.; private practice; Philadelphia

GRAY, Richard J., M.D.; Director, Surgical Cardiology; Cedars-Sinai Medical Center, Los Angeles

GROVER, Frederick L., M.D.; Chief, Cardiothoracic Surgery; Audie L. Murphy VA Hospital, San Antonio

HUTCHINSON, John E., III, M.D.; Chief, Cardiac Surgery; Hackensack Medical Center, New Jersey

KEAST, Marja-Leena; Physiotherapist; University of Ottawa Heart Institute Prevention and Rehabilitation Centre at the Ottawa Civic Hospital

KROZEK, Karen Sadler, R.N.; Cardiac Rehabilitation Nurse; St. John's Hospital and Health Center, Santa Monica, California

LAKS, Hillel, M.D.; Chief, Division of Cardiothoracic Surgery; UCLA Center for the Health Sciences, Los Angeles

LANDERS, Carole B., R.N.; Director, Cardiac Care & Diagnostic Center; Humana Heart Institute International, Louisville

LANSING, Allan M., M.D., Ph.D.; Chairman and Director; Humana Heart Institute International, Louisville

LUSK, Ruth, R.N.; Transplant Coordinator; Humana Heart Institute International, Louisville

MASRI, Zahi H., M.D.; Staff Surgeon; Humana Heart Institute International, Louisville

MATLOFF, Jack, M.D.; Director, Department of Thoracic and Cardiac Surgery; Cedars-Sinai Medical Center, Los Angeles

McCLURE, Albert L., R.N.; Clinical Coordinator; Humana Heart Institute International, Louisville

MOORE, Pam, R.N.; Director, Cardiovascular Services, Brotman Medical Center, Culver City, California

POLK, Jody; Accounts Manager, Cardiothoracic Group; UCLA Center for the Health Sciences, Los Angeles

RAHIMTOOLA, Shahbudin, M.D., M.B., F.R.C.P.; George C. Griffith Professor of Cardiology; Chief, Section of Cardiology; Professor of Medicine; University of Southern California School of Medicine and L.A. County/ USC Medical Center, Los Angeles

RESNEKOV, Leon, M.D.; Head, Department of Cardiology; University of Chicago Medical Center

ROBBINS, Bernie, M.S.W.; Social Worker; University of Ottawa Heart Institute Prevention and Rehabilitation Centre at the Ottawa Civic Hospital

ROBBINS, Patricia, R.N.; Cardiac Rehabilitation Nurse; University of Ottawa Heart Institute Prevention and Rehabilitation Centre at the Ottawa Civic Hospital

ROGERS, Sue; Clinical Dietitian, The Lipid Center; Humana Heart Institute International, Louisville

SCALLORN, Bobbie, R.N.; Cardiac Surgery Nurse Coordinator, Audie L. Murphy VA Hospital, San Antonio

SCHULMAN, Barbara, R.N., C.P.T.C.; Regional Organ Procurement Agency of Southern California

SHAH, Prediman K., M.D., F.A.C.C.; Director, Inpatient Cardiology and Cardiac Care Units; Co-Director, Fellowship Training Program, Cedars-Sinai Medical Center; Associate Professor of Medicine, UCLA School of Medicine, Los Angeles

SHAHEEN, Kevan A., R.N.; Manager, The Lipid Center; Humana Heart Institute International, Louisville

SNYDER, John; President; Mended Hearts, Kentuckiana Chapter No. 11, Louisville

STERTZER, Simon H., M.D.; Director of Medical Research; San Francisco Heart Institute, Seton Medical Center, South San Francisco

STRAKER, Manuel, M.D.; private practice (psychiatry); Los Angeles

STROBECK, John E., M.D.; private practice; Oakland, New Jersey

TEICHMAN, Sam L., M.D.; Director, Professional Services; Genentech, Daly City, California

TRINKLE, J. Kent, M.D.; Head, Division of Cardiothoracic Surgery; University of Texas Health Science Center, San Antonio

WEEKS, Ruby; member; Mended Hearts, Kentuckiana Chapter No. 11, Louisville

WIMSATT, Kim, R.N.; Clinical Coordinator; Humana Heart Institute International, Louisville

In addition, we cite the following publications by their single name or initials, as listed:

AHA—American Heart Association pamphlet "1988 Heart Facts"

LAT—Los Angeles Times

NYT—New York Times

HEART BEAT—(Horovitz, Emmanuel, M.D. (Health Trends Publications, Encino, CA 1988) (see page 112)

UCLA Manual—"Cardiac Transplant Teaching Manual," a guide for outpatient care

Page

3   larger numbers of women—Alpern, Resnekov

6   "Some patients"—DeVries

7   "standing with fingers crossed"—Teichman

     "drive the cholesterol level"—Goldburgh

     rehab program typically—Krozek, McClure

9   only the dimmest notion—adapted from *Survive*

10 fn   The full, formal name—word etymologies, passim, from *Webster's New International Dictionary*, Second Edition (G. & C. Merriam Co., Springfield, 1945)

11   beating about 100,000 times—AHA

     about 70% narrowed—HEART BEAT

     pain comes from a combination—Teichman

12   Irritation of heart tissue—Shah

     About 50% of deaths—AHA gives it as 60%, but Shah says it's closer to 50%

13   *Cardiomyopathy*—AHA, HEART BEAT

     Congestive Heart Failure—ibid.

     Heart Attack—adapted largely from *Survive*

14   patient can readily survive—McClure

     Valves—AHA, HEART BEAT

15   *All Have In Common*—*Survive*

     "People with coronary conditions"—Strobeck

17   Plaque has longer—Gibson, Moore, Strobeck

     "this area of the country"—Strobeck

     one therapist guesses—Gibson

18   never cholesterol we eat—HEART BEAT, UCLA Manual

     Cells make membranes, vitamin D—AHA

     more apt to develop—HEART BEAT

     "It's *important* to control"—Alpern

     work almost twice as hard—"Help Your Heart Eating Plan," pamphlet published by the American Heart Association in Texas

19   drawn convincing link—AHA

     "Two studies"—Alpern

     Stanford University study—LAT, 11/3/88

Page

19   men are still twice as likely—AHA

Guilty—except as noted, adapted from *Survive*

23   *High Blood Pressure*—Largely AHA, HEART BEAT

24   "If you don't control"—Alpern

"Smoking is clearly associated"—Alpern

damages the walls—HEART BEAT

smoking doubles the risk—AHA

"just crazy"—Grover

Ottawa . . . three months to quit—Dafoe, Keast

25   experiments with monkeys—Alpern

"integral part of life"—Rahimtoola

"dull people without some stress"—Landers

"people . . . thrive on stress"—HEART BEAT

"it signals to the family"—It was put another way by Dr. Alpern: "In dealing with families where a spouse has had a heart attack, younger members should be motivated by this to look at themselves. It's very important in any book addressing relatives of someone with heart disease: you have to learn what to do for yourselves and what to do for the children to prevent trouble in the future."

29   In cardiac catheterization—HEART BEAT

"one-tenth of 1%"—HEART BEAT cites a 1–2% rate of "major complications."

30   Guidelines—NYT, 8/1/88

31   standby surgical team—NYT, 8/2/88; LAT, 8/29/88, which reported that a hospital in Long Beach, California was forbidden to perform any further angioplasties because of their failure to provide for standby surgery

"thirty cases in 1000"—NYT 8/2/88: 3.5%

33   Not all arrhythmias require—HEART BEAT

underlying cause serious enough—Shah

34   close to 300,000 bypasses—NYT, 8/2/88

"better than vein grafts"—Cohn; NYT, 8/9/88

35   "The first thing we teach them"—Phillips quoting Holly Culley

one authority baldly puts it—HEART BEAT

one sufferer described—Phillips

Page

35   *Cholesterol*—general sources: LAT, 7/5/88, 11/15/88, 11/17/88; NYT, 7/21/88

push cholesterol level far enough down—Goldburgh

36   mechanics of cholesterol—AHA

HDL 25% of total—LAT, 1/31/89

falls below 35—Shaheen

37   American Medical Association symposium—LAT, 7/5/88

Clot Dissolvers—general sources: The Arizona Republic, 4/10/88; LAT, 4/13/88, 8/12/88, 11/16/88

"restore blood flow"—Teichman

38   "very exciting time"—Arizona Republic, *op. cit.*

difference . . . strep. and TPA?—Teichman, Arizona Republic, *op. cit.*

38 fn   Apsac—Arizona Republic, *op. cit.*

39   government boggled at price—LAT, 4/13/88

As in the old days—Brown

40   Thanks to sensitive tests—Strobeck

41   LVAD—except where noted, Frist

"back to the drawing board"—Masri

42   perform more bypasses as emergencies—Gray

Everyone in family should know . . . drugs—HEART BEAT

45   Lasers, for example—Stertzer; also NYT, 7/28/88

46   the Hemopump—Time Magazine, 6/16/88; NYT 8/1/88

Canadian researchers are developing—LAT, 12/12/88

the "stress-thallium" test—HEART BEAT

47   "a poor man's angiogram"—Gray

48   *Valves*—except where noted, Gray

only treatment for many years—HEART BEAT

50   Mr. P, a new patient—Phillips

51   20,000 and 30,000—DeVries

15,000—Laks (and colleague, Dr. Davis C. Drinkwater) in Western Journal of Medicine, November, 1988

"only" 10,000—Frist

52   patients find hard to grasp—Scallorn

Page

53   One medical group worried—Grover

Dr. Christiaan Barnard performed—USA 12/2/87

One of his nurses finds—Holly Culley, from Phillips

54   Forty-four states require—LAT, 8/2/88

56   "The ways things work"—Frist, from Phillips

average is around 40 days—Phillips

"I checked in at noon"—Phillips

59   relatively simple operation—Handbook for Transplant Recipients, University of Texas Health Sciences Center

flush it with ice-cold solution—NYT, 6/16/88

sending it to the lab—Teichman

59 fn   researchers in California—NYT, 6/16/88

60   "I was weaker than hell"—Phillips

61   77% of all recipients—Western Journal of Medicine

62   Q: How long in the hospital?—Phillips

Depending on your condition—Phillips

63   A lawyer in his late 30s—Phillips

transplant recipients "are sitting and watching"—Robbins

"I'm not certain"—Scallorn

64   At UCLA, which has outstanding record—Western Journal of Medicine

65   Transplant patients have given up—Scallorn

"people like Al and Jimmy"—Holly Culley, from Phillips

67   Better techniques in anesthesia—Gray

68   IS THIS PROCEDURE NECESSARY?—LAT, 12/27/88

doctors routinely order angioplasties—LAT, 11/16/88

outweigh charm and compatibility—As Dr. DeVries puts it, "The first conversation between the doctor and the patient and family ought to be: Will we get along? and am I going to have input about my desires, and is this the type of person that will care for me and nurture me? Or is this doctor's reputation so good that I don't care that he's a pain in the neck; I'm just going to lie down and do what he tells me and get well."

69   "Out of all the specialists"—Phillips

Is this a serious, difficult case—Teichman

71   The RAND Corporation . . . studied—LAT, 7/22/88

Page

73   *Doctors, Switching*—except as noted, from *Survive*

75   come *only* from examining doctors—*Survive*

77   How do they feel about—DeVries, Frist

      Finances and Insurance—largely, Polk

78    $100,000 transplant, etc.—Frist

80   insurance company recently announced—NYT 7/28/88

      1988 survey—LAT, 7/24/88

81   Another California survey—LAT, 12/27/88

84   *Children—Survive*

85   *Denial*—except as noted, *Survive*

86   "medical schools don't teach"—Brown

88   "doctor is not usually"—Rahimtoola

      reference to any registered dietitian—Rogers

      Studies show—McClure: "Several studies have shown that the
      patient who's well-prepared, pre-operatively, has a shorter hospital
      stay"; also, UCLA symposium, recorded by the authors

89   many patients forget—Scallorn

90   Oh! are you by yourself!—*Survive*

      The hardest thing is—Brown

91   "heart now as good as 18"—Snyder

      Clinical Coordinator . . . shocking—McClure

94   A nurse who deals—Holly Culley, from Phillips

      "Those kinds of things I *appreciate*"—Lusk

      chances are, no matter what (to end of section)—*Survive*

95   *Psychological Reaction*—except as noted, *Survive*

99   *Weaning Anxiety*—except as noted, *Survive*

99 fn endarterectomy—HEART TERMS, pamphlet published by the
       Department of Health, Education and Welfare

100   *Who Should Be Told*—except as noted, *Survive*

102   "can't tell a child absolutes"—Moore

104   *Atmosphere*—except as noted, *Survive*

106   "patient feel less dependent"—Grover

      "finding a way to argue"—Brown

      Doing Things—except as noted, *Survive*

Glossary

Adrenalin – Hormone produced by the adrenal gland that raises blood pressure and increases heart rate.

Aneurysm – A ballooning out of the wall of a blood vessel or a heart chamber due to a weakening of the wall by disease or injury.

Angina – Temporary pain when heart muscle receives too little blood to sustain its current level of activity.

Angiogram – X-ray movies taken of the heart and its arteries at work.

Angioplasty – Dilation of narrowed arteries by means of a balloon inserted in the artery and inflated at the point of narrowing, compressing the plaque that blocks the artery.

Anticoagulants – Drugs that slow down or prevent the blood clotting process.

Aorta – The large artery that carries blood from the heart's main pumping chamber (left ventricle) to the chest and abdomen.

Aortic Valve – Valve that passes oxygenated blood from the left ventricle to the aorta.

Arrhythmia – irregular heart beat.

Arteriosclerosis – Hardening and loss of elasticity of the arterial walls (commonly called "hardening of the arteries").

Artery – Blood vessel through which oxygenated blood flows from the heart to any other part of the body. The body contains many different arteries.

Atherosclerosis – Similar to arteriosclerosis; but in addition, plaque forms on the inner walls of the artery, causing an obstruction to the flow of blood.

Atrium (pl. atria) – One of the two upper chambers of the heart. The right atrium receives unoxygenated blood from the body. The left atrium receives oxygenated blood from the lungs. Both atria pump blood to their respective lower chambers (ventricles) during heart beat.

Beta Blockers – Medication that slows the heart and makes it contract less vigorously.

Blood Pool Scan – Diagnostic test that shows how the ventricle is beating by filling the heart chambers with a radioactive substance, allowing a picture of the heart motion.

Blood Pressure – Measure of the force exerted by blood against arterial walls as it is pumped by the heart.

Blood Vessels – Arteries and veins.

Bovine – From a cow or steer.

Bypass – See *Coronary Bypass Surgery*.

Calcium Channel Blockers – Medication that reduces coronary artery spasm by affecting calcium in the cells of heart tissue.

Cardiac Arrest – Cessation of heart beat.

Cardiac Output – Amount of blood pumped by the heart with each beat.

Cardiogenic Shock – Shock that results from damage to the heart.

Cardiomyopathy – Disease of the heart muscle in which the muscle stretches and weakens, or thickens, or hardens.

Cardiopulmonary – Pertaining to the heart and those blood vessels going to the lungs.

Cardiovascular – Pertaining to the heart and any blood vessels.

Cardioversion – Shocking the heart with a small amount of electricity to stop arrhythmias, allowing normal cardiac rhythms to continue.

Catheterization – General: insertion of thin tube (catheter) into body; Coronary: insertion into artery or vein (in groin or arm), with catheter directed into the heart for the purpose of examining heart function.

Cholesterol – Fatty substance found in the blood; it is manufactured from fats in the liver.

Coagulation – Clotting of blood.

Collateral Circulation – Process by which smaller vessels take blood to tissue that was fed by the artery now blocked.

Congestive Heart Failure – Accumulation of fluid in lungs and other body tissue due to impaired beating of the heart.

Coronary Bypass Surgery – Technique of grafting a length of vein or artery from a point above the blockage of a coronary artery to a point below the blockage, restoring blood flow through that artery.

Defibrillation – Like cardioversion—for a specific, common kind of arrhythmia.

Digitalis – Drug that strengthens heart contraction and slows the rate of beating, relieving buildup of fluid in body tissues.

Dilation – Stretching, widening, enlarging.

EKG – See *Electrocardiography.*

Echocardiography – Use of sound waves to show the structure of the heart motion and speed of blood in the heart chambers.

Edema – Swelling.

Effusion – Accumulation of fluid between body tissues or in body cavities.

Electrocardiography (ECG, EKG) – Diagnostic technique to record electrical activity of the heart with small metal discs placed on the chest, arms, and legs.

Embolism – Blocking of a blood vessel by a clot or other substance in the blood stream.

Fibrillation – Uncoordinated contractions of individual heart muscle fibers resulting in irregular heart beat.

HDL – See *High-density Lipoprotein.*

Heart Lung Machine – Apparatus that takes over pumping and cleansing function of heart and lungs during heart surgery.

High-density Lipoprotein – Type of cholesterol that carries other types away from arterial walls; so-called "good cholesterol."

Holter – Portable EKG recorder that permits monitoring for 24 hours while patient pursues normal activities.

Hydrogenated – Fat processed so that it solidifies at room temperature.

Hypertension – Condition characterized by excessive pressure within one's arteries.

Idiopathic – Of unknown cause.

Infarction – See *Myocardial Infarction.*

Intraaortic Pump – Pump inserted into the aorta, helping pump blood, thereby lessening the work the heart must do.

Invasive – Entering the body.

Ischemia – Decreased blood flow to tissue.

LDL – See *Low-density Lipoprotein.*

LVAD – See *Left Ventricular Assist Device.*

Laser – Beam of light; in coronary care, used to destroy arterial plaque, often in conjunction with angioplasty.

Left Ventricular Assist Device – Pump inserted in the left ventricle to take over part or all of that chamber's pumping duties.

Lesion – Injury; any morbid change.

Low-density Lipoprotein – Type of cholesterol that carries other types to arterial walls; so-called "bad cholesterol."

Lumen – Opening, specifically of a blood vessel through which blood flows.

Mammary Arteries – Arteries from the aorta to the breast region; sometimes used in coronary bypass surgery instead of vein graft.

METs – Measure of amount of energy expended for a given activity (metabolic equivalents).

Mitral Insufficiency – Leakage of the mitral valve causing back flow of blood in the wrong direction between the left ventricle and left atrium.

Mitral Stenosis – Narrowing of the mitral valve opening, resulting in incomplete opening.

Mitral Valve – Valve regulating blood flow between the left atrium and left ventricle.

Morbid – Unhealthy.

Monounsaturated – Fat that lowers the amount of cholesterol in the blood stream slightly.

Myocardial Infarction – Irreversible damage to heart tissue (death of the tissue) as the result of total blockage of the blood supply.

Necrosis – Death (generally applied to tissue).

Nitrates – Drugs that relax and dilate walls of blood vessels, lowering blood pressure.

Nitroglycerin – Drug that relieves spasm in coronary arteries, widely used to treat angina.

Occlusion – Shutting off of a blood vessel by blockage of the opening.

PVC – See *Premature Ventricular Contraction.*

Pacemaker – Electrical device that substitutes for the sinus node, regulating the heart beat with small electric discharges; usually implanted in the chest.

Palpitation – Sensation of fluttering, or other abnormally fast rate or rhythm of heart beat.

Patency – Openness of a blood vessel.

Perfuse (Perfusion) – Supplying tissue with blood.

Premature Ventricular Contraction – Condition when the ventricle contracts by itself, before the atrium contracts, rather than in rhythm, after the atrium; results in interrupted blood flow.

Plaque – Growing clump of various kinds of cells at the site of damage to the wall of an artery; can eventually block artery.

Polyunsaturated – Fat that can reduce amount of cholesterol in blood stream.

Porcine – From a pig.

Pulmonary Artery – Large artery that carries unoxygenated blood from right ventricle to the lungs.

Reperfusion – Flooding tissue with blood after it has suffered ischemia.

Saturated Fat – Fat, solid at room temperature, that promotes formation of cholesterol in the blood stream.

Septum – Wall of muscle dividing the left and right sides of the heart.

Sinus Node – Group of cells in the right atrium that naturally regulates the rate and rhythm of heart beat with small electrical discharges.

Sphygmomanometer – Actual name of familiar cuff, bulb, and dial used to measure blood pressure.

ST Segment – One of the significant EKG measurements.

Stenosis – Narrowing.

Stents – Mechanical devices (often coils of wire) inserted in arteries after angioplasty to keep them open.

Streptokinase – Bacterial agent that dissolves blood clots.

Swan-Ganz Catheter – Catheter with a balloon tip used to monitor conditions from inside blood vessels and the heart.

TPA (or tPA) – See *Tissue Plasminogen Activator.*

Tachycardia – Abnormally fast heart beat.

Thallium Stress Test – Diagnostic procedure in which radioactive thallium dye is injected while patient exercises on treadmill; allows picture of blood flow through coronary arteries.

Thrombolytic – Tendency of blood to form clots.

Thrombosis – Formation of blood clot that partially or completely blocks vessel.

Tissue Plasminogen Activator (TPA) – Protein that dissolves blood clots.

Tricuspid Valve – Valve with three flaps (cusps) regulating blood flow between right atrium and right ventricle.

Triglyceride – Common type of fat found in the blood stream.

Vasodilator – Drug that dilates blood vessels.

Vena Cava – Large vein that brings unoxygenated blood to right atrium.

Ventricle – One of two lower chambers of the heart. Left ventricle pumps oxygenated blood through the arteries to the rest of the body; right ventricle pumps unoxygenated blood to the lungs for oxygenation.

Ventricular Fibrillation – Chaotic beating of the ventricles resulting in stoppage of blood flow.

Valvoplasty – Surgical repair of heart valves.

Wall Motion Scan – Diagnostic procedure using nuclear material to show how wall of the ventricle is contracting.

Xenograft – Heart transplant from nonhuman animal to human.

Index